W9-CVO-324

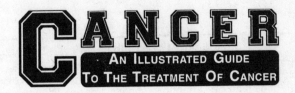

CANCER
AN ILLUSTRATED GUIDE
TO THE TREATMENT OF CANCER

Symptoms - Causes - Diagnosis - Surgery -
Diet - Homoeopathic Treatment

by

Dr. Harbans Singh Khaneja

To
Hona.
HON:

B. JAIN PUBLISHERS (P) LTD.
NEW DELHI

NOTE FROM THE PUBLISHERS

Any information given in this book is not intended to be taken as a replacement for medical advice. Any person with a condition requiring medical attention should consult a qualified practitioner or therapist.

CANCER

AN ILLUSTRATED GUIDE TO THE TREATMENT OF CANCER

© All rights are reserved. No part of this publication may be reproduced, stored in a retrieval system or transmitted, in any form or by any means, mechanical, photocopying, recording or otherwise, without prior written

1999 E
A

First Edition: 2002

Published by

KULDEEP JAIN

for

B. Jain Publishers (P) Ltd.

1921, Chuna Mandi, St. 10th, Paharganj,
New Delhi-110 055
Ph: 3670430, 3670572, 3683200, 3683300
Fax: 011-3610471 & 3683400
Website: www.bjainbooks.com, Email: bjain@vsnl.com

Printed in India by
Unisons Techno Financial Consultants (P) Ltd.
522, FIE, Patpar Ganj, Delhi-110 092

ISBN : 81-7021-1096-X
BOOK CODE : BK-5546

PREFACE

Today we are able to split an atom; but despite all the advances in medical research, cancer remains to be one of the most elusive and challenging disease to treat. Cancer is the second leading cause of death after heart diseases. One of the problems in fighting cancer is that cancerous cells can slip away from the original tumor and migrate throughout the body to other locations, creating secondary tumors called *Metastasis*. We have more knowledge, more experts and more medicines but less infirmity as far as cancer is concerned.

We constantly hear of new breakthrough in the worldwide compaign to find decisive cures for cancer. The latest conventional treatment is still rooted in the *holy trinity of surgery, chemotherapy and radiation*. The most prevalent conventional treatment "Chemotherapy" develops potentially serious side effects, particularly neutropenia (a low white cell count), fatigue, severe nausea, mouth sores, diarrhea, anemia, decreased platelet count and hair loss. Shocking reality is that cancer cases continue to rise each year. The exact causes of it are not known, but this has been associated with the following:-

1. Stress and anxiety.

2. Foods—Non vegetarians tend to develope cancers more than vegetarians.

3. Excessive tea and coffee drinking.

4. Alcoholic drinkers are at greater risk of developing cancers than the non alcoholics.

5. Smoking.

SIMPLE FOOD AND SIMPLE LIFE IS KEY TO GOOD HEALTH

A homoeopathic physician has to face many problems in selection of a remedy. Different medicines are required for different kinds of cancers and their location in the body. In the homoeopathic repertories, there are many medicines for one disease and also there is one remedy for many complaints. *Similarity of symptoms* should be the criteria for selecting an indicated remedy for this; the physician should have a thorough knowledge of materia medica from A to Z. According to the classical homoeopathy, common symptoms hold the least value and peculiar symptoms are of greatest importance. In evaluating symptoms one must keep in mind which ones are truly representative of the patient and which are marely common manifestations of the diagnostic category of the pathological entity. For example, a pain that is worsened by movements is a common symptom and is of little significance whereas the pain that is reduced by movements has greater relavance for homoeopathic prescription. There is no single remedy which can cure every case of cancer. Different remedies may be required at different stages. *It is important to remember that a homoeopath treats the whole person and not the disease alone.* This principle implies deciding what is the best remedy for each individual. The same treatment is not necessarily used for all people with the same disease.

The diagnosis of cancer must be made by the modern methods and laboratory investigation before starting the treatment. Many cases are erroneously diagnosed as cancer cases which, in fact, they are not. Wrong diagnosis can kill a patient. The physician should believe in his knowledge of remedies, diseases and human anatomy and treat the case with confidence. When the selected remedies do not produce relief, anti-miasmatic remedies like *Thuja, Medorrhinum, Syphilinum,* etc. should be employod to induce the system to respond to the proper remedy. Besides these, cancer nosodes like *Carcinocin* and *Scirrhinum* also vacate cancer miasms. Homoeopathic treatment can still prevent development of many cancers.

Treating cancer is not easy. It requires a skillful, educated and intelligent doctor. It is a wrong idea that all forms of cancers can be cured. Two cases of cancer are never alike and a thorough knowledge of materia medica is necessary. Symptoms should be given weight in every form of treatment. Each case must be studied *carefully* for selecting the leading and guiding symptoms for the indicated remedy or remedies. In my practice of homoeopathy, for the last more than 57 years, as compared to other diseases I have seen only a few cases of cancer—mostly the cases spoiled by faulty surgery or complicated cases in the terminal stages. Hence I cannot boast of my vast practical knowledge of the disease. Cancer is a traumatic event and a patient just turns off when told that he/she has a cancer. Knowledge is power and the more knowledgeable is a patient about the silent enemy that has invaded his/her body, the more powerful will be he/she to battle the disease. This book has been designed to give that knowledge. Various journals and medical books served as resourses for the purpose. The knowledge so gained is summerized and presented in a language that is easily understandable even by those without any medical knowledge.

The diseases and remedies have been arranged in an

alphabetical order for sake of convenience only and not in order of their importance.

I hope that this practical and illustrated guide which is a distillation and condensation of about 57 years of experience and studies will be found useful by cancer patients, medical professionals as well as general public.

HARBANS SINGH KHANEJA

3134 MERRITT AVENUE
MISSISSAUGA (ONT)
CANADA L4T-IP3

ACKNOWLEDGEMENT

The distillation and condensation of my 57 years of experience, studies and three years of writing of this researched book could not have been possible without the help from my wife Mrs. Harbans Kaur Khaneja who spared me from all the household worries and Dr. Jasleen Kaur Khaneja, DHMS (Gold Medalist), who typed this book and assisted me in my clinic work during this period. My profound thanks are due, to both of these ladies.

HARBANS SINGH KHANEJA

Contents

Chapter	Page no.
Cancer	1
Diagnostic tests	5
Bladder cancer	9
Blood cancer (leukemia)	15
Bone cancer	21
Brain tumor	25
Breast cancer	29
Colo-rectal cancer	37
Eye cancer	43
Face cancer	45
Heart cancer	47
Kidney cancer	49
Larynx cancer	53
Liver cancer	57
Lung cancer	59
Lupus	63
Lymphoma (hodgkin's disease) (lympho-sarcoma)	67
Mouth cancer	75
Myeloma	79
Nose cancer	83
Oral cancer (cancer of the lips, tongue, mouth and gums)	85
Ovarian cancer	89
Pancreatic cancer	93
Penis cancer	97
Prostate cancer	99

Scrotum cancer -- 103

Skin cancer and myeloma -------------------------------------- 105

Spinal cord cancer --- 111

Stomach cancer --- 115

Testicular cancer --- 121

Throat cancer--- 125

Thyroid cancer -- 127

Tongue cancer--- 131

Uterine cancer -- 133

Cancer of vagina --- 139

Cancer of vulva -- 141

Five steps to prevent cancers -------------------------------- 143

Tumors--- 147

Cancer pains-- 153

Sexuality and cancer -- 157

Allopathic treatment of cancer ------------------------------- 161

Hope for the future -- 165

Chapter-1

CANCER

Cancer is a disease in which abnormal cells in some organ or tissue go out of control, growing and increasing in number. Normal cells reproduce themselves throughout life, but in an orderly and controlled manner. Normal growth occurs, worn out tissues are replaced and wounds heal. When the cells grow out of control and form a mass, the mass is called a *Tumor*. Some tumors grow and enlarge only at the site where they began and they are called *Benign tumors*. Other tumors not only enlarge locally but have the potential to invade and destroy the normal tissues around them and to spread to distant parts of the body. Such tumors are called *Malignant Tumors* or *cancers*. Distant spread of a cancer occurs when malignant cells detach themselves from the original (primary) tumor and are carried to other parts of the body through blood or lymphatic vessels and establish themselves in the new site as an independent (secondary) cancer. A tumor which has spread in this manner is called metastasized and the *secondary tumor* or tumors are called metastasis or metastases. Cancer are represented by three great classes as below:-

1. Sarcoma: Such cancers arise from the underlying

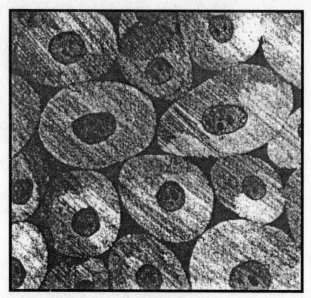

Normal cells

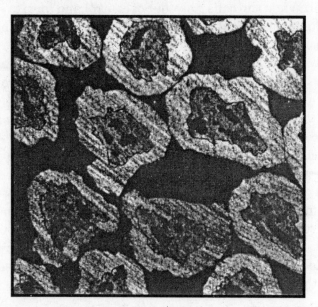

Cancer cells

tissues and these may effect bones.

2. **Carcinoma:** It is a malignant tumor enclosing epithelial cells in connective tissue and may affect any organ or part of the body.

3. **Lymphoma:** It affects vessels and organs of the body lymphatic system (spleen, thymus, lymph nodes).

Canadian statistics show 10 top cancers in canada during the year 2001 as listed below:-.

MEN	WOMEN
Prostate: 17800	Breast: 19500
Lung: 12100	Lung: 9200
Colorectal: 9300	Colorectal: 7900
Bladder: 3500	Uterus: 3500
Non-Hodgkin's Lymphomas: 3400	Non-Hodgkin's Lymphomas: 2800

SYMPTOMS OF THE CANCER

1. Unusual bleeding—external or internal.

2. A lump or sore which refuses to heal.

3. A change in bowel or bladder habits.

4. Hoarseness and persistant cough.

5. Indigestion or difficulty in swallowing.

6. A change in size or appearance of a wart.

7. An unexplained loss of weight.

NOTE : Cancer is not an easily treatable disease. It takes a very long period and several medicines.

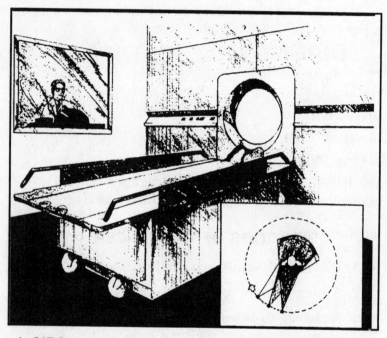

In CAT Scan, a computer directs X-ray beams from a rotating disc at regular intervals. The beams travel through the portion of the body being studied onto a device that registers the beam's findings. The results are analyzed by a computer, and the data appear as at three-dimensional image on TV screen.

Chapter-2

DIAGNOSTIC TESTS

The following procedures are generally adopted to diagnose a cancer.

BIOPSY

This test is done to determine whether the tumor is cancerous (malignant) or harmless (benign). A small piece of the tissue of the suspected area is removed and is examined under the microscope by a pathologist or an expert doctor.

BLOOD COUNTS

Samples of blood on a slide are examined under a microscope to determine the red cells and white cells count.

PLATELETS COUNT

Platelets are found in the blood of vertebras and play an important role in blood coagulation where there is an injury. This test is made in a given amount of blood to determine the disorders like *Thrombocytosis* (increased platelet count) that occurs after operation and *Thromb-*

ocytopenia (reduced platelet count) that occurs in acute infections. Platelets do not contain hemoglobin.

BONE MARROW TEST

Samples of bone marrow are taken by making tiny incisions in the hip area and this can leave the patient in a minor discomfort for a short time.

CAT SCAN (COMPUTERIZED AXIAL TOMOGRAPHY)

In this test, a computer directs X-ray beams from a rotating disc at regular intervals. The beams travel through the portion of the body being studied into a device that registers the beam's finding. The results are analysed by a computer and the data appears as a three dimensional image on a TV screen.

ECHOCARDIOGRAM

It helps in study of the functioning of the heart. It is an ultrasonic technique to produce a graph of the echo produced when the sound waves are reflected from the tissues of different density.

LUMBAR PUNCTURE

It is made to test the cerebrospinal fluid. Puncture is made by placing an aspiration needle into the sub-arachnoid space of the spinal cord and is usually done in the lumber area at the level of 4th intervertebral space.

MRI (MAGNETIC RESONANCE IMAGING)

This gives incredible snap shots of the body for detection of illness of the bone marrow, disorders of ligaments and cartilages and their injuries, detects tumors and nervous disorders.

MYELOGRAM

Roentgenographic inspection of the spinal cord by use of a radio-opaque medium injected into the intrathecal space. It is done to test the tiny lymphocytes formed abnormally in the bone marrow and tumor originating in the cells of homoeopoetic portion of the bone marrow.

RADIOISOTOPE STUDIES (SCANS)

ULTRASOUND STUDIES (ECHO STUDIES)

COLONOSCOPY

This is done to examine the lining of the large bowel to detect tumors or cysts. A long flexible tube (*Colonoscope*) about the thickness of a finger is inserted into the rectum and slowly advanced through the colon while the patient is lying on the left side. There is little pain and to make the patient comfortable, he is made sleepy by a medication. Air is used to inflate the bowel. The prcedure takes about 30-60 minutes. The condition of the bowel is displayed on a TV screen. It can be enlarged and photographed.

MAMMOGRAPHY
(ROENTGENOGRAPHIC STUDY)

This process involves obtaining pictures of the breasts by use of roentgen rays for diagnosis of cancer in them.

SIGMOIDOSCOPY

This is almost similar to colonoscopy. It is done to examine the sigmoid flexure of the colon i.e. lower part of the descending colon, between the iliac crest and the rectum shaped like the letter S. The test is done by a sigmoidoscope which is a tubular speculum.

PYELOGRAPHY (IVP)

It involves roentgenography of the renal pelvis and ureter by use of roentgen rays.

NEPHROTOMOGRAPHY

This is used for ascertaining renal tumor. Nephron is the structural and functional unit of the kidney. There are about one million nephrons in each kidney.

PAP TEST

This test is used for examination of the cervix to detect its cancer. The test is simple and takes only a few minutes. A speculum is inserted into the vagina upto the cervix. A small medical spatula and a tiny brush are then used to remove a few cells from the surface of the cervix for examination under the microscope.

Chapter-3

BLADDER CANCER

STRUCTURE

Bladder is a membranous sac or a recepticle and it acts as a reservoir of urine which it receives from the kidneys through the ureter and discharges it out from the body through the urethra. It is situated in the anterior portion of the pelvic cavity. In females, it lies in the front of the anterior wall of the vagina and uterus. In males, it lies in front of the rectum. More than 85% of all bladder cancers originate from the transitional epithelium.

SYMPTOMS

Usually the first and the only sign of the bladder cancer is *presence of blood in the urine.* Other symptoms include frequent urination, strong urges to urinate and discomfort or burning sensation during urination and involuntary leakage of urine—small or large. It is extremely rare in pregnancy. A burning pain with constant tenesmus and hemorrhage is a sure symptom for the disease.

CAUSES

Smoking is the major cause of the cancer of bladder. Other causes can be worry, meat eating, tea, coffee or alcoholic stimulants and injury to the bladder.

DIAGNOSTIC TESTS

X-rays of the bladder and visual examination of the bladder through a scope inserted through the urethra.

SURGERY

There are several methods of surgery for removal of the cancer of the bladder and most of them result in impotency in males and physiological changes like alteration in sensation and potential for orgasm in females. In *cystectomy*, the bladder, uterus, ovaries, fallopian tubes, cervix and uterus are all removed. This can create several problems.

DIET

Drinking about 2-3 litres of fluids like water, soda, etc. each day can cut the risk of bladder cancer to half. The liquids probably flush away carcinogens and keep the urine diluted so that the toxins can make less contact with the bladder wall.

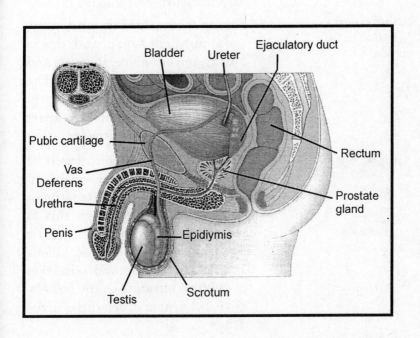

Bladder
Ureter
Ejaculatory duct
Pubic cartilage
Rectum
Vas Deferens
Prostate gland
Urethra
Penis
Epidiymis
Testis
Scrotum

HOMOEOPATHIC TREATMENT

CALENDULA Q : Has a remarkable power to reduce the cancer bleeding and removes bad odor of the bleeding if present. Give 10 drops doses twice daily as an inter-current remedy.

CHIMAPHILA UMBELLATA Q : Scanty urine loaded with ropy, muco-purulent sediment. Urine is bloody and offensive. Burning and scalding during micturation. The patient is unable to urinate without standing with feet wide apart and the body bent forward.

CHOLINUM Q : This remedy is a constituent of Taraxacum root. It has given encouraging results in the treatment of bladder cancer. When this is indicated, there are some gastric disturbances like headache, bilious attacks, flatulence and sensation of bubbles bursting in the bowels. Give 1-2 drams doses three times a day.

EQUISETUM Q : Severe dull burning pain and feeling of fullness of bladder not relieved by urinating. Frequent urging with severe pain at the close of urination. Urine flows only drop by drop. Dose 15 drops once in two hours.

EUCALYPTUS Q : Hematuria. Urine contains pus. Bladder feels loss of expulsive power. Burning and tenesmus. The cancer is small and fleshy.

EUPHORBIUM 30C : It is a palliative for reducing burning pains of the cancer and periodical cramps.

TARAXACUM Q : Cancer of bladder with sensation of bubbles bursting in the bowels. Modalities are better by touch on the region of bladder and are worse lying down and resting. Dose 2 drams BDS.

TEREBINTHINA 6C : Five drops of it - once in two hours relieves tenesmus, burning pains and bleeding. There is constant distress in the bladder as if it is overfilled with urine.

THUJA 200 : A dose may be given before commencement of the treatment with the indicated remedy.

LEUKEMIA

WHERE IS IT FOUND ?
THE BLOOD

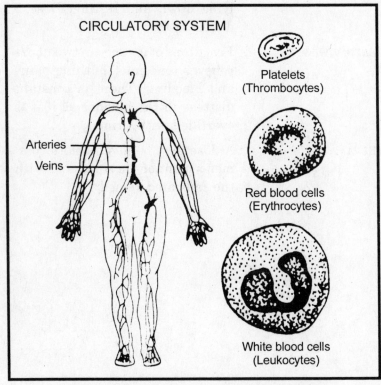

CIRCULATORY SYSTEM

Platelets
(Thrombocytes)

Red blood cells
(Erythrocytes)

White blood cells
(Leukocytes)

Arteries

Veins

Cells not shown in actual proportion to one another

Chapter-4

BLOOD CANCER (LEUKEMIA)

STRUCTURE

Leukemia literally translated means white blood which suggests a condition characterised by immensely increased numbers of abnormal white cells in the blood. The basic abnormality lies in the blood forming tissues, the bone marrow and lymph nodes. There is no tumor. Instead immature white cells proliferate in the bone marrow which previously produced only normal, healthy cells. The immune cells continue to multiply in the bone marrow and eventually spread into the blood. As the number of abnormal cells increases, the number of normal cells decreases. Decreased number of red cells and platelets leave the patient anemic and susceptible to infections and bleeding. There are four types of leukemia:-

1. **Acute Lymphoblastic Leukemia:** This predominantly attacks children though it can occur at any age.

2. **Acute Myeloblastic Leukemia:** This commonly appears in adults.

3. **Chronic Myelocytic Leukemia:** It commonly occurs in mid life. It can also be found in teenagers and

older patients.

4. Chronic Lymphocytic Leukemia: It seldom appears in patients under the age of 40.

SYMPTOMS

Blood samples reveal high white cells count and their immaturity; and decrease of red cells and platelet counts. Other symptoms include fatigue, loss of weight and enlarged lymph nodes in the neck and groin.

CAUSES

Till today no cause or causes of this disease have been identified other than high doses of radiation or previous chemotherapy. Compelling evidence comes from high number of people who developed leukemia following explosion of atomic bomb at Hiroshima, Japan. Viruses do not cause this disease.

DIAGNOSTIC TESTS

Microscopic examination of the blood and bone marrow. A sample of blood is drawn from the vein and red and white cells are counted. Any deviation is confirmed by biopsy of the bone marrow. Examination is made under a microscope.

SURGERY

Surgical and radiotherapeutic treatment, common therapies in most cancers, are infrequently used to treat. On occasions, lymph nodes and spleen may be surgically removed. If a patient is not cured in this way, bone marrow is transplanted from a related donor,who must be a close relative. New technologies involve autologous transplants (where patients receive their own marrow after its cure), peripheral stem cells transplant and fetal cord blood transplants.

DIET

Simple vegetarian diet and eating of 5-10 servings of vegetables and fruits a day. Avoiding alcoholic drinks and smoking.

HOMOEOPATHIC TREATMENT

ARSENICUM IODATUM : All discharges are corrosive and acidic and mostly watery and fetid.

ARSENICUM HYDROGENISATUM 6 : Dr. Raymond Warell, a leukemia specialist at Memorial Sloan-Kettening Cancer Centre, New York (USA) found low doses of arsenic extremely effective in treatment of this disease without any side effects. The characteristic symptoms include restlessness in the afternoon and midnight, debility, shortness of breath, weak heart action and palelessness of the face. Gradual loss of weight. Swollen feeling of parts. General blood deorganization.

BARYTA MURIATICA 3X : Vertigo, increased tension of pulse and high systolic pressure with comparatively low diastolic pressure. Cardiac symptoms are usually present.

BENZINUM 6 : Increase production of white blood cells and decrease production of R.B.C.

CALCAREA CARBONICA	: Sweating of head. Swelling of cervical and inguinal glands. Remittent fever.
CALCAREA PHOSPHORICA:	Mostly indicated in children who are peevish, fretful, lean and feel better in summer.
CEANOTHUS Q	: Splenomegaly, pain in the spleen and violent dyspnea are guiding symptoms. 5 drops a dose three times a day.
CHINA	: Dislike for mental or physical exertion. Swollen and hard liver. Enlarged spleen with pain. Skin is hot and dry. Fever is marked with periodicity and chills.
CHININUM SULPHURICUM	: A rapid decrease in red blood cells and hemoglobin with a tendency to polynucleate and irregular white cells.
FERRUM PICRICUM 3X	: Useful for symptoms like leukemia i.e. pseudoleukemia.
MERCURIUS SOLUBILIS 200	: Its use decreases the high count of white blood corpuscles.
NATRIUM SULPHURICUM 6X	: Desires ice or ice cold water. Splenic and lymphatic leukemia. Pale face. Piercing pain in extremities. Suits severe cases of the disease.
PSORINUM	: Phagocytes are defective. Patient is chilly, weak and always very hungry.

RADIUM BROMATUM	: This remedy may prove useful when there is a marked increase in the white blood cells having more than one nucleus.
THIOSINAMINUM	: It is a remedy for wasting of spinal marrow and should prove useful in this disease.
VANADIUM METALLICUM 6	: It is a carrier of oxygen. Increases the amount of hemoglobin and stimulates the function of white blood corpuscles (phagocytes).

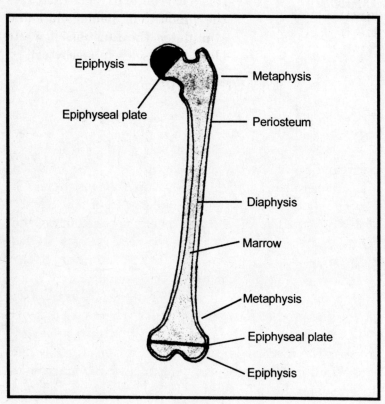

Bone

Chapter-5

BONE CANCER

STRUCTURE

Enveloped in the body's soft tissues, the human skeleton, in most people, consists of 206 bones. This supports the body and protects vital organs such as the heart, lungs and brain. It also produces several types of blood cells. Bones are not lifeless. Rather, they are dynamic structures capable of growth. Two layers of elastic connective tissue, the periosteum, cover the bone but not the joints. A network of blood vessels and nerves weave through the outer layer and also the interior cavity or the marrow to provide its nutrients. Certain hormones, minerals such as calcium and phosphorus and bone cells control the process of wear and tear by replacing it with new bone tissue. Diseases can alter and interfere in this process. The marrow is concentrated in the ribs, breast bone, skull, pelvis and spine. The spongy red marrow is the site of production of red cells, most of the white blood cells and platelets.

SYMPTOMS

Pain of the bone tumors is often felt in the knee,

thigh, upper arms, ribs and pelvis. These are the bones where tumors generally develop. Pains are worse at night. Depending upon the type of cancer, the patient may have fever, night sweats and weight loss. The bones affected by sarcoma cause swelling around them and the flesh becomes hard and immovable.

CAUSES

To date, the precise cause of bone cancer is not known. It is suspected that in some adolescents and adults the hormonal changes linked with rapid bone increase may increase the risk of osteosarcoma. Exposure to high doses of radiation during childhood may cause osteosarcoma, chondrosarcoma and fibrosarcoma in later years. Sarcoma generally develops at the site of the injured or fractured bone.

DIAGNOSTIC TESTS

Regular X-rays, CAT scan, Radioisotope Scan, MRI and biopsy.

SURGERY

For small osteosarcoma and chondrosarcoma in the legs or arms, the tumor is totally removed along with one or two inches of normal bone and the soft tissues surrounding it. The bone is replaced by a piece of suitable bone or by a metal prosthesis. If the tumor is large, the entire bone is removed without amputating the limb. Chemotherapy treatment is also given, if required.

DIET

Variety of simple vegetarian foods and milk 2%.

HOMOEOPATHIC TREATMENT

AURUM IODATUM 3X : The mucous membrane is always red, swollen, itches and burns. Night sweats.

AURUM METALLICUM 30C : Nightly pains are important indication for the use of this remedy. Soreness is better in open air. The patient is hopeless and has suicidal tendencies. Cancer of the closed cavities of bones.

CALCAREA FLUORICA 12X : Osteosarcoma of tibia bone of the leg. Bony (osseous) tumors on the neck or back and encysted tumors on the back of wrist. The result of use of this remedy is known after a few days and then it should not be repeated too soon.

HECLA LAVA 3X : It is a useful remedy in the sarcoma of bones. It repairs bones, tissues and surrounding areas destroyed by the disease.

PHOSPHORUS 30C : Cancer heals and return again at the same site. Pain is better by washing with cold water and is worse by warm foods and warm drinks.

PHYTOLACCA Q : It helps growth of fibrous and bony tissues after healing of the bone cancer.

SYMPHYTUM Q : Its use stimulates the growth of epithelium and helps heal the bone. Cancer of peristeuneum of the bones with irritation of bones.

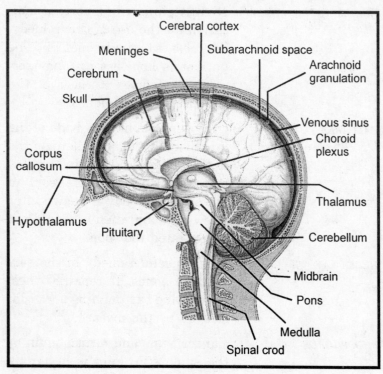

Cerebral cortex

Meninges

Subarachnoid space

Cerebrum

Arachnoid granulation

Skull

Venous sinus

Choroid plexus

Corpus callosum

Thalamus

Hypothalamus

Cerebellum

Pituitary

Midbrain

Pons

Medulla

Spinal crod

Brain

Chapter-6

BRAIN TUMOR

STRUCTURE

An organ which regulates all the functions essential for   an active life.

SYMPTOMS

General symptoms of brain tumor are headache and vomiting   without   nausea.   The vision is also affected. *Neuroblastoma* is the rare and lethal cancer of the nervous system. It originates in the embryonic neural cells in the neck, chest, abdomen or pelvis. It may be present at birth but may not produce any symptom. Mental changes, dullness, epileptic convulsions and giddiness are other signs. Such tumors do not contain any blood vessels but may produce pain and other sensations.

CAUSES

Exact cause is not known uptill now. It may be hereditary.

DIAGNOSTIC TESTS

1. **Cranial X-ray pictures:** Air is injected into the ventricles prior to the X-ray examination. The examination is known as *Pneumo-ventriculography.*
2. **Nuclear Magnetic Resonance (EEG)**
3. **Biopsy**

SURGERY

The operation performed on the brain is called *Craniotomy*. During this procedure, a piece of the skull bone is cut away to expose the brain area where the tumor is growing. After the tumor is removed, the piece of bone is usually replaced, except when the brain tissue is very swollen. Most types of brain tumors have a tendency to swell and surgical intervention sometimes increases the amount of fluid in the tissues.

HOMOEOPATHIC TREATMENT

CALCAREA CARBONICA 200 : Tumor of brain. Headache and vertigo on turning the head. Icy coldness of the head. Tumors with roots.

CALCAREA FLUORICA 200: A very useful remedy when the tumor is hard and stony. Creaking noise in the head. Great depression. Sparks before the eyes. Brain fag and vomiting.

PLUMBUM METALLICUM : Epileptic form of convulsions, giddiness and in some cases coma. Pain as if ball rose from throat to the brain. Voices in the ears. This is a leading remedy.

SCIRRHINUM 1000	: A dose may be given at the start of the treatment. No medicine should be given for next 48 hours.
SULPHUR 200	: It should be used as an intercurrent remedy once a month and no medicine should be given for the next 24 hours.
THUJA 200	: Brain tumor with migraine headache. Flatulence. Constipation. The patient is emotional and sentimental.

NOTE: Malignant glimas and meningiomas, the most common types of the brain tumors, are aggressive, invasive and resistant to treatment. Most patients die quickly and long-term survival is rare.

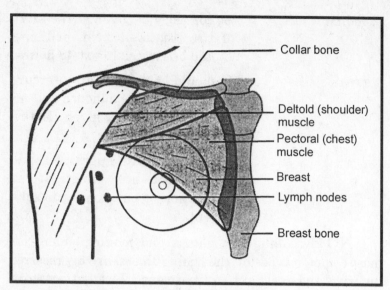

Breast

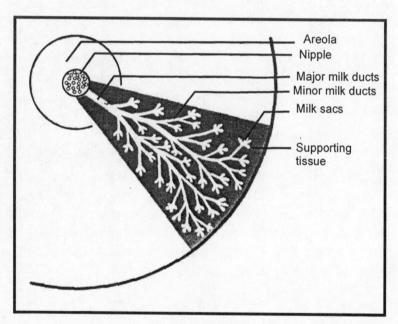

Breasts

Chapter-7

BREAST CANCER

STRUCTURE

Breasts are glandular (secreting) organs and are designed to produce milk. Each breasts contains 15-20 segments (lobes) and duct of each lobe opens seperately on the nipple. Breast tumors usually arise from the cells of milk sacs (ducts) although malignant tumors may occasionally arise from the supporting structure of the breast.

SYMPTOMS

Early sign of breast cancer is bleeding from the nipple. Alternately, it may grow into a mass which is usually very hard but in some cases it can be soft. The mass is mostly painless. This type of cancer is 100 times more common in women than in the men and becomes more common after the age of 50 years. It can spread to bones.

CAUSES

Causes of breast cancer are not yet known. The use of female sex hormone (estrogen) for a long time is con-

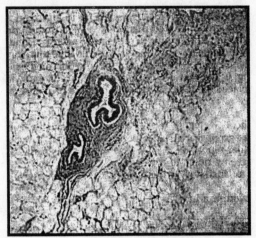

Normal Breast

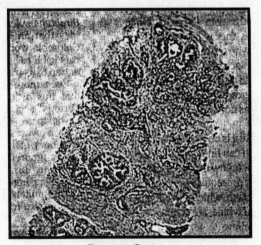

Breast Cancer

sidered one of the probable cause. There is no evidence to support that a breast cancer is caused by injuries to the breast.

DIAGNOSTIC TESTS

Mammography that is roentgenographic study, is used to diagnose the cancer. In this process the picture of the breast is obtained by use of roentgen rays.

SURGERY

The most common surgical procedures are:-

1. **Lumpectomy:** It involves removal of the tumor with bit of the adjoining normal breast plus the lymph glands of the armpit.

2. **Modified radical mastectomy:** It involves removal of the entire breast and tissues of the armpit.

3. **Radiation therapy:** This is increasingly being used.

4. **Chemotherapy:** It involves not only the destruction of cancer cells but also the normal cells.

DIET

In India, where the diet is often vegetarian there are less cases of developing cancer than in the Western and American World where people are mostly meat eaters.

HOMOEOPATHIC TREATMENT

APIS MELLIFICA 30 C : Cancer pain is burning and stinging. The breast is indurated.

ARSENICUM IODATUM 3X: The cancer is indurated, painful and sensative to touch. The glands in the axillae are swollen, hard and of the size of a walnut. Cancer of breast when ulceration has started.

ASTERIAS RUBENS 30C : Ulcerative stage of the cancer. Breast is hard and painful. The patient has red face. It acts on both the breasts but better on the left. The patient is fleshy. There is lancinating pain in the breast.

BARYTA IODATA 3X : It is useful when the cancer is hard and long standing.

BELLADONNA 200C : It is useful only when the disease is not prolonged. Breasts feel heavy, hard, hot and red and the pain is worse from lying down.

BELLIS PERENNIS Q : If the breast cancer has been caused by an injury or a blow or a bite, this is a remedy in the early stages of cancer.

BROMIUM 3C : Tumor with stitching pains which extend to axillae. Acts better on the left breast. Breasts are hard.

BRYONIA ALBA 30C : The lymphatic glands under the lower jaw are stony hard and pain in the breasts on little movement.

BUFO RANA 30C : Acts as a palliative in the breast cancer. Menses are clotty, too early and too profuse. Watery leucorrhea. Burning in the ovaries and uterus. Bloody milk.

CALCAREA FLUORICA 6X : The lump in the breast is hard and stony. The cancer may have spread to the bones. There is a stabbing pain, like the thrust of a needle.

CARBO ANIMALIS : Use it when the tumor is only in the nipple of the breast.

CARCINOSIN 200C : This fluid extract of specifically breast cancer is very useful in treatment of breast cancer. There is great pain and hardness of breast. One dose a week.

CHIMAPHILA Q : Tumor is painful. Breast is very large and nipple may be secreting undue milk or blood.

CONDURANGO Q : Cancer of breast with ulcers in the corners of the mouth or cramping pains in the stomach.

CONIUM MACULATUM 3X : Tumor is stony hard with burning and stinging pains. Breasts swell up at the time of menstruation.

CONIUM 1000C : Use it sparingly for the tumor in the left breast.

HECLA LAVA 3X : It repairs bones and tissues damaged by operation of breast.

HOANG NAN Q : 10-15 drops of tincture three times a day gives good results and removes the fetid odor; if cancer is bleeding; and revives healing process.

HYDRASTIS CANADENSIS 3X : Breast cancer is accompanied by constipation and distress in the abdomen after meals. Lancinating pain in the breast.

KALIUM MURIATICUM 6X	: A lump in the breast with a nodulated feeling accompained with a pain now and then. There may not be any discharge of blood from the nipple which may not be retracted. Axillary glands are not affected. Bunches in the breast feel quite soft and tender.
LACHESIS 200C	: Cancer of left breast which develops a purplish appearance. It bleeds easily and the blood is decomposed. Bleeding relieves pain and suffering.
PHYTOLACCA Q	: Very useful for treatment of secondary tumor (metastasis) of the breast. The breast is hard, painful and very sensitive to touch. It has a purple hue. Axillary glands are enlarged. The menses are too copious and too frequent. Give 5 drops once in 3 hours.
SCROPHULARIA NODOSA Q	: Ten drops in little water taken 3 times a day gives results in about 2 months.
SILICEA 6X	: When pus has formed in the cancer give 5 drops in warm water three times a day. There are lumps in the breasts which suppurate and discharge thick yellow offensive pus.
TARENTULA CUBENSIS 30C	: Cancer of breasts of very old ladies.
THYROIDINUM 2X	: Fibroid tumor of the breasts.

TUBERCULINUM 1000C   : Benign tumor of breasts.

NOTE: Breast cancers are somewhat linked to the ovarian troubles in many cases. Therefore treatment of the ovary and menses leads to the cure of the breast cancer. About 30% of breast cancer are rooted in the uterus or ovaries.

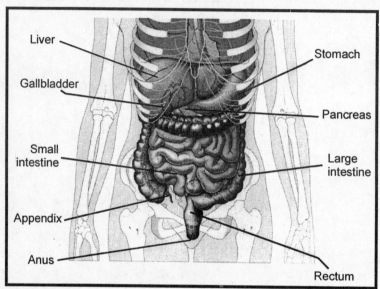

Liver

Gallbladder

Small
intestine

Appendix

Anus

Stomach

Pancreas

Large
intestine

Rectum

Digestive system

Chapter-8

COLO-RECTAL CANCER

STRUCTURE

Cancer of colon and rectum is called colo-rectal cancer. The colon, also called large bowel, is 5 to 6 feet of intestine. The rectum is the last 5 to 6 inches at the end of the colon, leading to the outside of the body. It is the leading cause of death after lung cancer. It can have all the characteristics of cancers in general. This tumor usually arises from the epithelial cells and on rare occasions , malignant tumor may arise from the supporting tissue. Cancer of colon is more common in men.

SYMPTOMS

A change of bowel movements which can contain bloody stools, or black tarry movements, diarrhea or constipation, nausea and abdominal pains. Bleeding from the rectum.

CAUSES

Following are the possible causes of colorectal cancer.The exact cause or causes have not yet been determined:-

1. Chronic ulcerative colitis.

2. Familial polyposis coli—a rare disease that occurs in many members of the same family and begins as a result of multiple benign tumors of the intestines.

3. *Large number of polyps* develop in the colon and rectum and overtime becomes cancerous. It is believed that every cancer starts from a benign polyp.

4. A strong history of colorectal cancer.

5. Consumption of too much of fats derived from the animal sources.

DIAGNOSTIC TESTS

Colorectal cancer is detected by the following tests:-

1. Rectal examination.

2. Test for occult blood in the stool.

3. Sigmoidoscopy: This is similar to the colonoscopy.

4. Colonoscopy: During this test, a portion of the infected area is removed for biopsy.

5. Barium X-ray.

6. General blood test.

SURGERY

Laparoscopic surgery is still the most commonly used treatment. Removal of a portion of diseased colon does not produce any serious after effects but surgery of rectum is a complicated affair. If the sphincter has to be removed along with the tumor, an outlet for the stool is made in the outside of the abdomen and a plastic bag is attached to it where the stool is discharged. Such an artificial opening is called *colostomy*. Radiotherapy or radiation therapy is used in combination with surgery and chemotherapy.

DIET

Simple leafy vegetarian foods and lot of water. A balanced, low fat and high fibre diet. Foods containing Vitamin C and E may help in protection against cancer in this area.

HOMOEOPATHIC TREATMENT

CARDUUS MARIANUS Q : Diarrhea due to the cancer of rectum.

CHININUM ARSENICOSUM 3X : Diarrhea painless, watery; very offensive stools and emaciation. Burning in the rectum.

COLOCYNTH 3OC : Cancer of sigmoid with lancinating pain shooting out through the bowels.

CONIUM : Trembling and sudden loss of strength while walking. Sever ache in the abdomen. Frequent urge to pass stools which are hard. Weakness is felt after each stool. Heat and burning in the rectum during defecation.

HYDRASTIS SULPHURICUM 30C : Hemorrhage of cancer of bowels. Smarting pain in the rectum during defecation.

HYDROCOTYLE ASIATICA Q : A useful remedy for treatment of rectal cancer and reducing its pain.

NITRIC ACIDUM 200C : Rectum feels torn. Constipation. On straining, a little stool passes. Bleeding from lower bowel.

NUPHAR LUTEUM 2X : Early morning diarrhea. The patient has to run to the toilet fearing that if not attended immediately, the stool may escape.

ORNITHOGALUM
UMBELLATUM Q

: Cancer of caecum and appendix with great debility. Vomiting of coffee-ground looking matter and a lump in the abdomen in the affected area. Depression and great prostration.

PHYTOLACCA Q

: 5 drops in half a cup of water, three times a day may absorb cancerous tumors of the rectum.

PODOPHYLLUM 3OC

: Constipation is frequently a great obstacle in giving relief to these patients. Give this remedy four times a day with a gap of 3 hours between two doses.

RUTA 3OC

: Carcinoma affecting the lower bowel with feeling of extreme weakness and despair. Constipation alternating with mucous diarrhea. Frequent unsuccessful urging to stools.

SEPIA 200C

: Feeling of presence of a ball in the rectum. Constant oozing from the anus. Bleeding at stools and fullness of rectum. Constipation. Large hard stools appearing like dark brown round balls glued together. Pain in the abdomen is better by drawing limbs up.

SPIGELIA 3OC

: Cancer of sigmoid flexure of colon with burning and unbearable pain.

STRYCHINE *SULPHURICUM 30C*	: Cancer of rectum. Tension and irritation in rectum. Pulse weak. Diarrhea bloody.
THUJA 200C	: Loss of appetite. Bloody diarrhea. Flatulence in the abdomen. Burning pains in the anus. Fungus growths and cauliflower type of cancer which has not ulcerated.

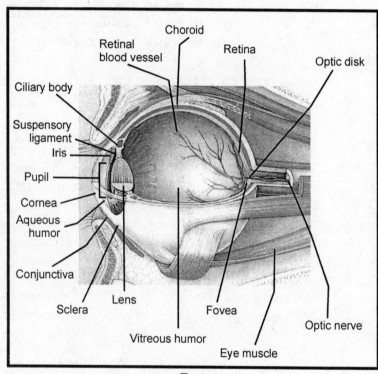

Eye

Chapter-9

EYE CANCER

STRUCTURE

Eye is composed of three layers— sclera, iris and retina. Anterior part of sclera forms transparent cornea behind which there is a lens. The cavity behind the lens is filled with a jelly-like substance. Light entering the eye passes through the cornea, then through the pupil it passes through the lens and jelly like substance and is incident upon the retina which has nerve endings which receive the impulse generated by the light. The sensory impulses are then conveyed to the brain which registers them as visual sensation.

SYMPTOMS

Eyes grow larger and become more prominent. Weakening eye sight. Pain in the eyes—headache. Little sparks before the eyes. The cancer may result in the blindness.

CAUSES

One of the causes is *Retinoblastoma*—a malignant tumor of the retina which is usually of hereditary pattern. It occurs in childhood. Causes of other cancer of eyes have not yet been discovered.

HOMOEOPATHIC TREATMENT

MORPHINUM 3X : Cancer of eyes causing dropping of lids. Delusion of vision on closing of eyes and partial paralysis of the lids. Look unsteady.

PHYTOLACCA : Ulcerated cancer near the eye which is spreading and has a considerable discharge. Apply it on the diseased parts. It dissolves the cancer and heals it.

ZINC SULPHATE 1M : A dose a month when the lids are granular and the vision is diminished.

Chapter-10

FACE CANCER

STRUCTURE

Anterior part of the head from forehead to the chin. It does not include ears. There are 14 bones in the face.

SYMPTOMS

A sore with oozing of pus on the face that refuses to heal with the routine treatment and when the ulceration continues with fetid discharge. Open sore with a scab constantly forming on the sore.

HOMOEOPATHIC TREATMENT

KALIUM SULPHURICUM 3X
: A small epithelioma of the face with scabs and a red angry appearance. There is thin yellow discharge.

LOBELIA ERINUS 30C
: Malignant tumor and carcinoma of the face and cheeks.

PHYTOLACCA Q
: 5 drops in water every 3 hours. It has a powerful effect when the cancer is accompanied with unex-

plained loss of weight.

STRYCHNINUM SULPHURICUM 3X : A dose every three hour can be given when there is over irritability, restlessness and cramps like pain.

Chapter-11

HEART CANCER

STRUCTURE

Heart is a hollow muscular contractile organ, and it is the centre of the circulatory system of the blood. It has three layers—the outer epicardium (a serous layer), the middle myocardium (composed of cardiac muscle) and the inner endocardium (a layer which lines the four chambers of the heart and covers the valves). It is enclosed in a fibrous sac, the pericardium. Heart functions day and night throughout life.

SYMPTOMS

Heart is not an easy area to look at and by the time a cancer develops in it, a lot of other problems appear in other parts of the body. Thus the heart cancer goes unnoticed due to the troubles so developed and the actual symptoms of the heart cancer become hard to detect.

CAUSES

The heart can develop primary cancer in any of its layers i.e. the lining of the heart or heart muscle itself or the fibrous sac in which the heart lies. It can develop secondary cancer or metastasis from a distant spread of malignant cells detached from the other cancerous parts of the body and carried through blood to it. Such cells establish in the new site in the heart. All the blood in the body flows through heart and as such heart should be a potential lodging site of a cancer and actually metastasis of the heart should be more common.

TREATMENT

Cancer in the various parts of the body like lungs, kidneys, liver, skin, etc. and their treatment has been discussed in this book. During my practice of homoeopathy for last about 57 years, I did not come across or ever heard of a case of heart cancer. According to Dr. Charles Catton (Radiation Encologist) of Princess Margret Hospital, Toronto which is a Premier cancer institute, a case or two of primary heart cancer turn up a year. Consultation of several homoeopathic books and reperteries did not reveal a treatment of heart cancer. This is a rarest cancer and perhaps no homoeopathic treatment has been discovered so far.

Chapter-12

KIDNEY CANCER

STRUCTURE

The two kidneys are located-one below the liver and the other below the stomach on either side of the spine. They filter wastes from the blood stream and discharge them from the body in shape of urine. The most common type of kidney cancer originates in the epithelial cell lining the renal tubules. It can spread usually through the blood stream and the lymphatic system. A few types of kidney cancer arise in the kidney's pelvis (the sac forming the upper part of the ureter) and these resemble the bladder cancer. Fibrosarcoma is the rare type of kidney cancer that develops in the renal capsule (the fibrous and fatty web encasing the kidney).

SYMPTOMS

The early sign of the kidney cancer are blood in the urine (hematuria) and the later symptoms include a pain or a lump in the kidney region. Transverse or perpendicular fissure on the tongue.

CAUSES

Smoking cigarrettes, pipe and cigars is strongly associated with developing kidney cancer. Even the smoke arising from burning of coal can give rise to this type of cancer.

DIAGNOSTIC TESTS

Usual tests to detect it are:-
1. Intravenous pyelography (IVP)
2. Nephrotomography
3. Computerized Axial Tomography (CAT Scan)
4. Ultrasound
5. Selected Renal Arteriography
6. Biopsy
7. Bone scan
8. Magnetic Resonance Imaging (MRI)

SURGERY

The procedure is called *nephrectomy*. In this procedure, the affected kidney, portions of the surrounding tissue and nearby lymph glands are removed. The other kidney takes up the functions of the kidney so removed.

HOMOEOPATHIC TREATMENT

CROTALUS HORRIDUS 6C: Cancer of kidney with great prostration and yellow color of the body skin. Fever and hematuria of dark fluid that forms no clots may accompany. More right sided in its action.

NOTE: Wilm's tumor accounts for 90 % of kidney cancer of children below 4 years of age.

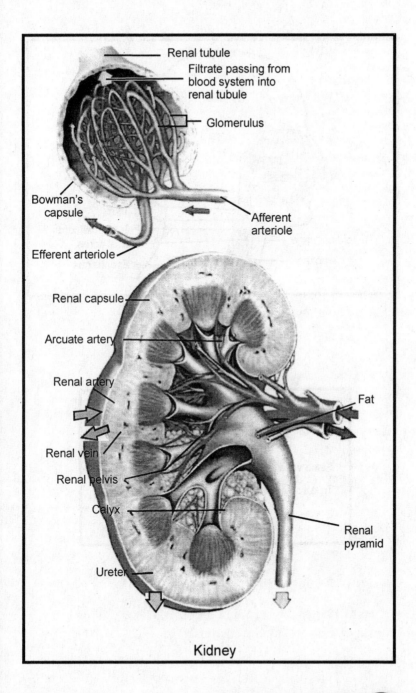

Renal tubule

Filtrate passing from blood system into renal tubule

Glomerulus

Bowman's capsule

Afferent arteriole

Efferent arteriole

Renal capsule

Arcuate artery

Renal artery

Fat

Renal vein

Renal pelvis

Calyx

Renal pyramid

Ureter

Kidney

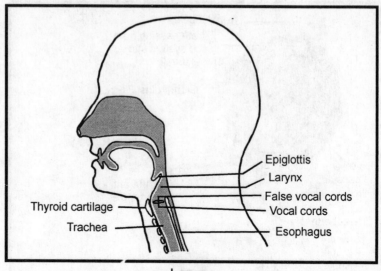

Larynx

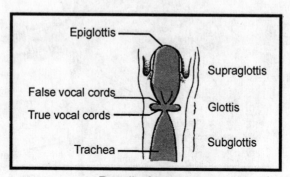

Detail of Larynx

Chapter-13

LARYNX CANCER

STRUCTURE

Resembling a box like chamber, the larynx is situated just below the chin in the neck and is connected to the trachea (windpipe). Its outside walls are formed by nine cartilages and inside of the walls is lined with a mucous membrane. Protuding from its top, is a flap like valve called epiglottis which prevents the food and liquids from entering the larynx and trachea. True vocal cords are mounted on U-shaped cartilages in it. When sound enters the mouth, it is formed into words by shape of the mouth and the position of tongue.

SYMPTOMS

Laryngeal cancer can develop in any part of the larynx but mostly it occurs in glottis area. Early tumor appears as an irregular ulcer on the vocal cord and as it progresses it spreads to the other cord. It rarely spreads to the neck except in its most advance stages. It can also develop in supraglottis area and in about half of the cases such a tumor can spread to the nearby lymph nodes and is carried to the other parts of the body. *Persistant hoarse-*

ness is *the first sign and it is followed* by *pain and trouble in swallowing*. If it is not treated early, earache in one ear and spitting of blood can also occur.

CAUSES

The most important cause of larynx cancer is smoking. The risk is substantially greater when the people smoke and drink together. Loud and constant use of voice can also cause it.

DIAGNOSTIC TESTS

Larynx can be examined by using a laryngeal mirror. In advanced cases, a long narrow flexible tube is threaded through the nose into the back of the throat. At the end of the tube is a light which illuminates the vocal cords. This quick procedure is called *"Fiberoptic Laryngoscopy"*. In microlaryngscopy, a tiny microscope attached to the tube magnifies the images of the vocal cords to detect the tumor. CAT Scan and Biopsy can actually diagnose the trouble.

SURGERY

In surgery, either all or part of the larynx is removed. When only a portion is removed, the patient retains his ability to speak though the sound may be somewhat altered. Such patients can breath and eat as before the operation. When total larynx removed, an opening called " Stoma" is made in the lower part of the neck to enable the patient to breath, cough and sneeze. Such a patient can eat and drink as before the surgery and with training learns to speak again. Chemotherapy is often used in the conventional treatment.

HOMOEOPATHIC TREATMENT

ARSENIC ALBUM 30C : Bloody saliva. Tongue dry, clean and red. Dryness and burning in the throat in the region of larynx; relieved by gulping very hot water. Throat appears constricted and there is inability in swallowing.

ARSENIC IODIDE 30X : Great emaciation. Burning in the region of the larynx and pharynx. Fetid breath. Otitis of one ear with fetid corrosive discharge. Dry cough.

CONIUM 30C : Bloody discharge from one ear. Continuous dry cough caused by dry spot in larynx and itching. Cough is worse when talking and laughing. Oppressed breathing. Raw feeling in the back of the throat when inspiring.

PHYTOLACCA 200C : Decrease of weight. Much pain in the region of larynx and the root of tongue. Shooting pain in the ears on swallowing. Cannot swallow anything hot. Dry hacking tickling cough worse at night.

SANGUINARIA NITRICUM 30C : Smarting and burning in the region of the larynx with a sense of obstruction and burning in the throat. Throat is rough, dry and difficult swallowing.

THUJA : Papilloma of the larynx.

Chapter-14

LIVER CANCER

STRUCTURE

Liver is the largest organ of the body and is situated on the right side of the abdomen beneath the diaphragm. Its secretes bile and has many metabolic functions.

SYMPTOMS

Severe pain and tenderness, loss of flesh and strength, enlargement of liver and jaundice may indicate the primary growth of a tumor. The disease is usually found in persons past the mid-age. The patient constantly presses his hand over the liver region to support as he walks.

CAUSES

Malignancy in the liver is as a result of spread from the primary source. Liver is the most usual site of metastatic spread of cancers through the blood stream. Liver cancer arising from the bile ducts is said to be the cause of many deaths.

DIAGNOSTIC TEST

Diagnosis is made by the test common to the test of

tumors in pancreas, etc.

SURGERY

Usual methods as in cancers of the glands in the abdomen.

HOMOEOPATHIC TREATMENT

CARDUUS MARIANUS Q : It reduces pain of the cancer of the liver and its inflammation and also the profuse diarrhea due to it. Give 10 drops a dose three times a day.

CHELIDONIUM Q : Perpendicular enlargement of the liver. A dusky color of the face. Constipation, indigestion and strong odor in the urine. Five drops three times a day.

CHOLESTERINUM 3X : Liver cancer with enlargement of the liver and burning pains in the liver region. Movements are painful; the patient has to hold his hand on the liver when walking. Jaundice. Emaciation. Yellow conjunctiva.

HYDRASTIS 6C : Cancer of liver before ulceration sets in when the pain is the main symptom. Emaciation, prostration, constipation and distress in bowels. Flatulence.

IODIUM 3X : Loss of flesh with great appetite. Always hungry, eats well yet becomes weak and lean. Liver is enlarged and is sore. Jaundice.

Chapter-15

LUNG CANCER

STRUCTURE

Lungs are two cone shaped spongy organs of respiration and are contained within the pleural cavity of the thorax. They are connected with pharynx through trachea and larynx. The base rests on the diaphragm. The primary purpose of the lungs is to bring air and blood into intimate contact so that oxygen can be added to the blood and carbon dioxide can be removed. *Adenosarcoma* usually arise from outer areas of the lungs. Cancer may appear in trachea, air sacs and other lung tubes. It may appear as an ulcer in the windpipe, a nodule or small flattened lump blocking the air tubes. It may invade surface of tubes and extend to lymphatics and blood vessels. About 40-45% of lung cancers are squamous cell cancers.

SYMPTOMS

This cancer, even well advanced, produces no outward symptoms. Cough is the most common symptom and it may also trigger shortness of breath and wheezing. Cough can be taken as ordinary symptom and this is why treatment is delayed. By the time, lung cancer is found the patient is nearly dead.

CAUSES

About 80 % of lung cancers are produced by smoking. Sometimes coal tar and asbestos products can also produce it. Smoking causes lung cancer in two ways. First of all smoke inhalation damages the normal cleaning process by which the lung protects itself from the injury. Bronchi—tube like structure, conduct inhaled air to the lung tissues. Hair-like cilia beat in rhythmic fashion to move the mucous membranes continually upwards from the lung, removing any inhaled particles trapped in the sticky mucus. Smoking makes the cilia to disappear and the lung lining thickens to protect the underlying delicate tissues from damage. On account of these changes, the lung cannot keep itself clean. Consequently cancer producing agents in the cigarrette smoke have their way. A person who has smoked for about 20 years is at the maximum risk of this type of cancer. Smoking includes passive smoking. Passive smoke contains carbon- monoxide, ammonia and nitrosamines. All of them are harmful to the lungs.

DIAGNOSTIC TESTS

1. **Examination of sputum** under the microscope.

2. **Bronchoscopic examination** of the airways is done by passing a tube through the mouth or nose into the airways subdivision of each lung. If an obstructing tumor is seen, its biopsy is done.

3. **Needle biopsy:** When the cancer cannot be detected by test no. 2 a fine needle is introduced through the chest wall directly into the tumor with the help of X-

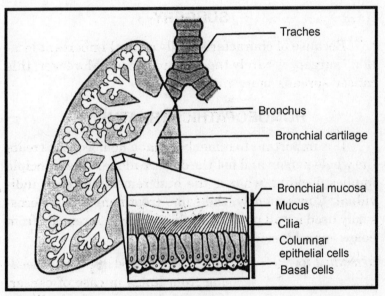

Lung

ray guidance. A small sample is taken out for biopsy.

4. **Mediastinoscopy:** To establish the case correctly in this test a tube is passed through an incision downwards alongside the airways to inspect the lymph nodes near the lungs. If abnormality is observed, biopsies can be obtained for examination.

5. **CAT Scan.**

SURGERY

Because of characteristically central important location, surgery is rarely the best treatment. Moreover, this cancer spreads more rapidly.

HOMOEOPATHIC TREATMENT

It is important to remenber that a homoeopath treats the whole person and not the disease alone. This principle implies deciding what is the best remedy for each individual. Consequently, the same treatment is not necessarily used for all people with lung cancer. A remedy from below may be selected in each case.

GERANIUM MAC Q : Vomiting of blood due to the bleeding from lungs in case of cancer. Give 20 drops every hour till the bleeding stops.

HIPPOZAENIUM 30C : Cancer of lungs with hoarseness and feeling of suffocation. Cough with much secretion of mucus. Irregular and noisy breathing.

NOTE: Smoking and alcohol consumption are the main causes of the lung cancer. This cause should be eradicated to eradicate the disease. Prevention is the best cure.

Chapter-16

LUPUS

STRUCTURE

This is a form of epithelial cancer and is also called *"Eating Cancer"*.

SYMPTOMS

It *first appears on the nose as a hard, dusky red sore* and spreads in ulcerative form destroying the tissues till the bones are exposed. This affects women 10 times more than men. It usually appears in women between the age of 20-40 years, although it can occur at any age. Nausea, vomiting and abdominal pain may accompany. It is an ulcerative skin disease and requires a very long-term treatment. Sensitivity to sunlight is usually present.

CAUSES

Lupus is caused by disruption of body waste disposal system from failure of special enzyme *"D-Nasil"*, which fails to remove wastes from the body.

DIAGNOSTIC TESTS

The disease is easily noticeable as it is outside the body on the skin and biopsy is performed to confirm it.

SURGERY

If possible, the affected portion of the body is cut out.

HOMOEOPATHIC TREATMENT

ALUMINA : Pale face. Blue lips with lupus on the nose.

APIS MELLIFICA : Lupus with characteristic effect like stings of the bees with rosy swelling and stinging pains and intolerance of heat and slightest touch.

AURUM MURIATICUM 3X : If the bones of the nose seem to be involved and there is very offensive discharge from the nose.

BACILLINUM 200 : The treatment should be started with this remedy and the indicated remedy should be given after seven days.

CISTUS : Lupus with hard and indurated glands.Skin hard, dry, fissured with deep cracks. Itching all over. Can be used locally in tincture 5 drops in one ounce of water to wash and arrest the fetid discharge.

GRAPHITES 200C : Lupus of nose when there is obstruction of the nares, cracked skin and every injury tends to ulceration. A dose every four days.

GUAREA Q	: Lupus with red, yellow or brown pigmentation of the skin. Yellow spot on the temple.
HYDRASTIS Q	: Lupus. Ulceration of the skin with thick yellowish ropy secretion. It should be applied locally mixed with glycerine in the ratio 1:3.
HYDROCOTYLE Q	: Dry eruptions with great thickening of the epidermoid layer &exfoliation of scales. Lupus without ulceration. There is profuse perspiration. A dose of 10 drops every three hour arrests the disease in a short time.
KALIUM BICHROMICUM	: Papular or vesicular eruptions resembling small pox with itching and burning.
RADIUM BROMATUM	: Inflammation and swelling of the skin with ulceration & redness. Burning of skin and itching.A good remedy under these circumstances for lupus.
SCROPHULARIA Q	: A valuable remedy in cases of lupus ulceration. It can also be painted on the affected parts.
STAPHYSAGRIA 6X	: This is a useful remedy in lupus where there are ulcers inside or outside the nose with bruised pain in the arm and legs.
THUJA 1000	: Treatment may be started with this remedy. Next indicated remedy be given after 24 hours of its

use. In some cases, use of this remedy alone in 30/c potency for a very long period may cure the disease.

Chapter-17

LYMPHOMA (HODGKIN'S DISEASE) (LYMPHO-SARCOMA)

STRUCTURE

It is a disease of special type of lymphoma or abnormal growth of cells in the lymphatic system, which is a network of small vessels called lymphatics which resemble the veins. It contains lymphatic fluid collected from the body tissues and carries it to the blood stream. It is a part of body's defence system. Lymphatic tissue is found in most organs of the body particularly spleen, liver, bone marrow and intestines. Along the course of lymphatic system are lymph nodes located throughout the body. Hodgkin's disease usually starts in the lymph nodes and can spread throughout the body involving lungs, abdominal organs and bones. Abnormal white cells multiply to increase 90% leaving a fewer white cells to fight the infection.

SYMPTOMS

Painless swelling of the lymph nodes in the neck, underarms or groin, sometimes nausea or vomiting or abdominal pain and diarrhea, persistant fever of un-

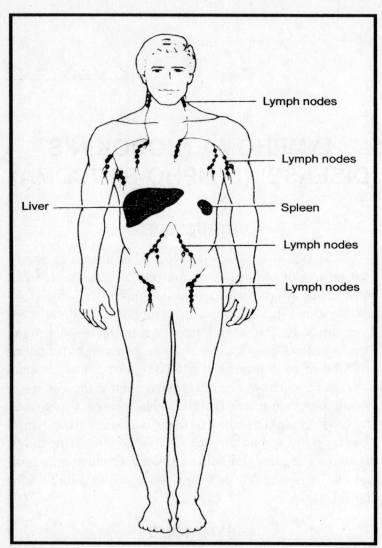

Lymphatic system

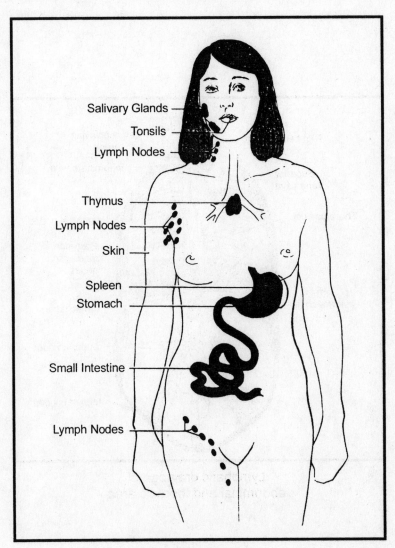

Salivary Glands
Tonsils
Lymph Nodes

Thymus
Lymph Nodes
Skin

Spleen
Stomach

Small Intestine

Lymph Nodes

Hodghkin disease

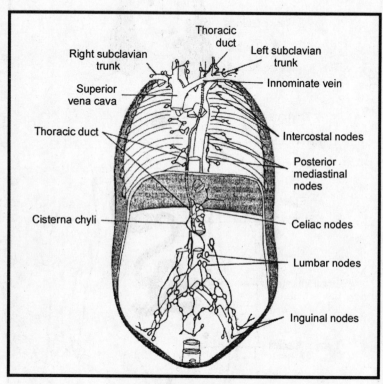

Lymphatic drainage of
abdominal and thoracic area

known cause, profuse drenching night sweats, unexplained loss of weight and shortage of breath. Enlargement of the lymphoid tissues, spleen, liver with invasion of other tissues.

CAUSES

Lymph nodes filter the lymph and remove disease-forming materials including cancer cells and sometime they become the site of cancer themselves.

DIAGNOSTIC TESTS

Biopsy, chest X-rays, blood tests, lymphangiography and Gallium scan.

TREATMENT

1. **Radiotherapy:** High energy X-rays or cobalt radiation is directed to the affected area to destroy or damage the cancer cells but leaving the surrounding tissues largely unharmed.

2. **Chemotherapy.**

Both the treatments cause some unpleasent side effects like nausea, vomiting, feeling of fatigue and hair loss.

DIET

Variety of lower fat, high fibre foods. Avoid smoking and alcohol.

HOMOEOPATHIC TREATMENT

ARSENIC ALBUM 30 : Gradual unexplained loss of weight and debility. It will maintain the system affected by the hodgkin's disease and in most of cases does not allow the disease to progress. Restlessness, afternoon and midnight aggravation.

ARSENIC IODIDE 3X : It covers symptoms like debility, watery diarrhea, recurrent fever, drenching night sweats, chilliness, etc.

CALCAREA CARBONICA 30C : Enlargement of lymphatic glands especially the cervical glands.

CEANOTHUS Q : 5 drops a dose three to four times a day is specific for enlargement of spleen resulting in anemia.

CHINA 30C : Periodicity of fever and chill with enlargement of the spleen. Change in bowel habits. Hot and dry skin.

CORYDALIS FORMOSA Q : In advanced cases of swollen lymphatic glands. There are dry scaly scabs on the face and there are symptoms of ill state of health as in case of old persons. Give 20 drops three times a day.

ECHINACEA Q : To ease pain in the last stages of cancers. It has a positive action on the immune system and helps production and increase of healthy white cells.

FERRUM PHOS 3X : Anemia and general debility.

HIPPOZAENINUM 30C : Cancer of lymphatic system. Swollen nodules in armpits and arms.

IODUM 3X : Cancer of lymphatic system with enlarged lymphatic glands. It arouses the defensive apparatus of the system to modify and clear leucocytes which are not normal. There is a very good appetite but inspite of it the patient gets thin and emaciated.

LAPIS ALBUM 6C : Enlargement and induration of glands of the neck, spleen, etc. The hardness is not much but glands retain certain amount of elasticity.

MERCURIUS SOLUBILIS 2X : This remedy affects all the lymphatic system with all the membranes and glands, internal organs, bones, etc. It's use produces good results provided the prescription is guided according to the symptoms of the remedy.

NATRIUM SULPHURICUM 6X : Liver enlarged. The patient cannot bear tight clothing around waist. Early morning diarrhea. Great size of the stool. Swelling of axillary glands, suits severe cases.

SCROPHULARIA MARYLANDICA Q : Cancer of the lymphatic system in advanced stages when there are lumps in the neck and axilla. In such cases, it is a splendid remedy. Dose 5 drops in a cup of water three times a day.

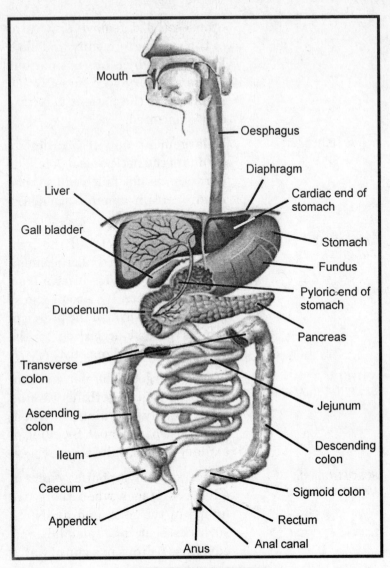

Mouth

Oesphagus

Diaphragm

Cardiac end of stomach

Liver

Stomach

Gall bladder

Fundus

Pyloric end of stomach

Duodenum

Pancreas

Transverse colon

Ascending colon

Jejunum

Ileum

Descending colon

Caecum

Sigmoid colon

Appendix

Rectum

Anus

Anal canal

DIGESTIVE SYSTEM

Chapter-18

MOUTH CANCER

STRUCTURE

Mouth is a cavity within the cheeks, containing the tongue, teeth and communicating with the pharynx. Cancer of the mouth is usually on the inside of the cheek or on the roof of mouth. Ninety to ninety-five percent of all oral cancers arise from the flattened squamous cells that line the mouth's soft tissues and are known as squamous cell carcinomas. Most of the sores, lumps, red or white patches seen or felt in the mouth or around the lips are not cancerous. They can be caused by cheek or tongue biting or dentures.

SYMPTOMS

1. Pain

2. Ulcers that do not heal.

3. Sore or wart-like eruptions on the lips.

4. Persistant sore throat.

5. A lump on the neck.

6. Difficulty in chewing or swallowing.

AN ILLUSTRATED GUIDE **75**

CAUSES

The vast majority of oral cancers perhaps 70-75% are caused by heavy smoking, combination of regular alcoholic consumption with heavy smoking. Repeated exposure to sunlight may cause cancer of the lower lip. Rarely, longtime irritation by the jagged teeth can also cause it. It does not spread by kissing or physical contact from a person to person.

DIAGNOSTIC TESTS

In addition to the visual examination, careful digital examination is made to reveal areas of alterations of texture characteristic of cancer. Lymph nodes are examined to see whether or not the cancer has spread.

SURGERY

Some oral cancers are removed by surgery and when it is performed, nearby lymph nodes in the neck are sometimes taken out as well.

HOMOEOPATHIC TREATMENT

CHROMIC ACIDUM 3X : Post nasal tumors and epithelioma of the tongue are benefitted by use of this remedy.

HECLA LAVA 3X : This remedy is useful in bony, hard tumors of the jaw. Give four doses in a day.

NITRIC ACIDUM 3X : Pain and swelling of the jaw, especially the upper one with hardness. A dose three times a day.

OXALIS ACETOSELLA JUICE : The dehydrated thickened juice is used to remove cancerous growth of the lips.

SEMPERVIVUM TECTORUM Q	: Scrirhous induration of the tongue. Carcinoma of cheeks and malignant ulcers in the mouth. Whole mouth is very tender.
SILICEA 6X	: A raised, firm, thickened red scar which has grown for a prolonged period of time and may have made a hole through the cheek outside on the face.

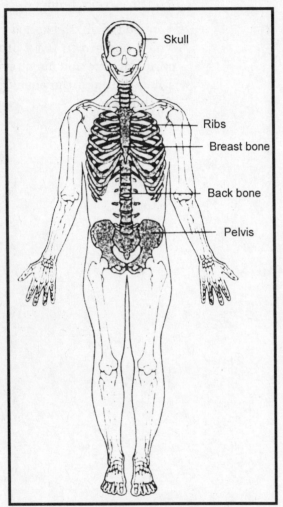

Multiple myeloma

Chapter-19

MYELOMA

STRUCTURE

It is *a neoplastic disease characterized by infiltration of bone and bone marrow by myeloma cells forming multiple tumor masses.* The plasma, a type of white blood cells undergo a malignant change and begin to multiply rapidly. The disease is more common in males than females in the ratio 3 : 1. *Plasmocytic sarcoma* is common in over 60 year of life. It is progressive. Plasma cells are rarely found in the blood stream of healthy persons but when body is invaded by infectious agents, plasma cells fight it. Plasma cells ocassionally form solid tumors and move from bone marrow to one bone and through the blood to the other marrow.

SYMPTOMS

Myeloma can be a new growth or an existing growth and has several appearances, including a skin growth or a sore that does not heal, an unusual lump, a rough red spot. Anemia, renal lesions and high globulin levels in blood. Bone pains, fatigue, abnormal bleeding, repeated infections and gradual loss of weight.

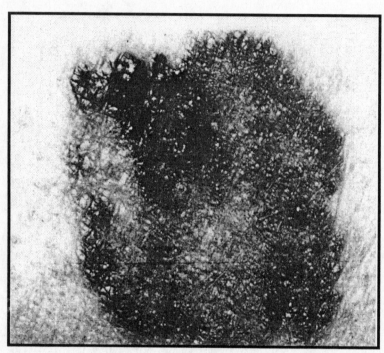

Melanoma

CAUSES

Red or blond hair, suppressed immune system, family history of skin cancer. Chronic exposure to some industrial toxin, sunburns and sun exposure, moles, high fat diet. Exposure to X-rays are the main risk factors of myeloma. Exact cause of this disease is still unknown.

DIAGNOSTIC TESTS

Microscopic examination of the suspect cells by a pathologist or dermatologist and biopsy.

SURGERY

1. **Electro-desiccation** (tissue destruction by heat).

2. **Cryosurgery** (tissue destruction by freezing).

3. **Radiation** (destroying cancer with rays that produce minimal damage to the surrounding normal tissues).

DIET

Vitamin A helps to fight this disease.

HOMOEOPATHIC TREATMENT

ARSENIC 3C-200 : Cancer arising from overgrowth of fibrous tissues or a cancer originating from the epidermis of the skin—may be hard or soft. Start the treatment with 3C potency and give it four times a day and go on selecting the potency which effects the most. If this remedy cannot cure, it will atleast reduce the pain and maintain or restore the general health.

CANNABIS SATIVA Q	: Fatty acids found in hemp protect the skin against sun. 15 drops in half a cup of water is used for protection of the skin against the skin cancer due to the sun rays.
EUPHORBIUM 6C	: Ulcerating carcinoma and epithelioma of the skin.
HYDRASTIS 30C	: Cancerous formation on the skin. Skin is ulcerated with smallpox like eruptions.
KALIUM ARSENIC 30C	: Skin cancer with no other visible symptoms except many small nodules under the sun.
LOBELIA ERINUS 30C	: Epithelioma, that is malignant tumor consisting principally of epithelial cells and originating from the epidermis of the skin or in a mucous membrane and developing rapidly. Dryness of the skin, nose and mucous membrane of the cheeks.
RADIUM BROM	: Cancer of skin with itching, burning and restlessness. Epithelioma.

NOTE : Multiple myeloma is marked by overgrowth and malfunction of plasma cells in the bone marrow. *It is amongest the most deadly and difficult to treat* cancer and it rarely yeilds to treatment.

Chapter-20

NOSE CANCER

STRUCTURE

Nose is the external portion and projection in the centre of the face. Its function is to act as an entrance of air and to warm, moisten and filter it for its entry into the respiratory tract.

SYMPTOMS

Offensive discharge from the nose. Reduction of opening of nares with difficulty in breathing.

CAUSES

A chronic ulcer, polyp or cyst.

DIAGNOSTIC TESTS

Nosochthonography. Lymph nodes are examined to see whether or not the cancer has spread.

HOMOEOPATHIC TREATMENT

CHROMICUM ACIDUM 3X : Post-nasal tumors with bloody foul smelling discharge. Scabs in the nose. Offensive smell.

LOBELIA ERINUS Q	: Carcinoma of epidermis of the skin or mucous membranes of the nose. Locally, it is antidotal to the cancerous germs.
PHYTOLACCA Q	: Give internally 10 drops a dose thrice daily and paint it externally four times a day for sarcoma of the nose.
SCROPHULARIA Q	: It is a valuable remedy in treatment of sarcoma on the external nose. Internally 10 drops a dose thrice daily and apply it mixed with glycerine in the ratio 1:3 thrice daily. It may cause disappearance of the cancer.
TRIFOLIUM PRATENSE Q	: Cancer of the external or internal nose with dry scaly crusts.

Chapter-21

ORAL CANCER (CANCER OF THE LIPS, TONGUE, MOUTH AND GUMS)

STRUCTURE

Frequent seats of oral cancer are lower lip, the tongue, the floor of the mouth and the gums. Less frequently it can also appear near the tonsils, salivary glands and on the soft tissues lining the cheeks. If not treated early, cancer cells spread to the neck, lymph nodes and jaw bones.

SYMPTOMS

This cancer can be easily detected by a sore and a swelling in the mouth and a lump in the neck. Most sores, lumps, red or white patches in the mouth or on the lips are not cancerous as these can be caused by tongue biting. In advance stages, there can be trouble in speaking, in chewing and in swallowing.

CAUSES

Research has shown that oral cancer affects people

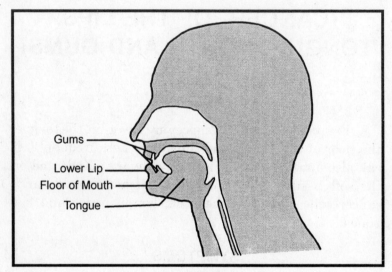

Gums

Lower Lip

Floor of Mouth

Tongue

Oral Cancer

who smoke or chew tobacco or betal nuts for long periods. Drinking of large amounts of alcoholic beverges and direct exposure to strong sunlight's ultraviolet rays can also be the possible causes.

DIAGNOSTIC TESTS

Biopsy is performed on the suspected areas to confirm the cancer.

TREATMENT

Radiotherapy is commonly used in the treatment. It damages or destroys the cancer cells while minimally affecting the surrounding normal tissues. The lymph nodes of the neck are removed.

DIET

The causes as referred above should be avoided and easily chewable vegetarian diets should be preferred.

HOMOEOPATHIC TREATMENT

ARSENIC IODIDE 3X : Epithelioma of the lips which is painful.

OXALIS ACETOSELLA JUICE : Fresh juice of the plant applied locally on the cancerous growths of the lips destroy the cancer.

PHYTOLACCA : Blisters on the sides of the mouth with a fissure or a yellowish patch in the middle of the lip. Pain in the lips during rains or exposure to cold and damp weather.

SEPIA 6X : In epithelial cancer upon the lip which bleeds often and has a broad base with burning pain, pricking as from a needle.

STRYCHNINE SULPHURICUM 30C : This remedy should be given three times a day with a gap of three hours between two doses in cases of oral cancer.

Chapter-22

OVARIAN CANCER

STRUCTURE

Ovaries resemble in shape and size with an almond and are situated in the pelvic region—one on either side of uterus, behind and below the fallopian tubes (See illustrations). There are three types of ovarian cancer: *Epithelial, germ cell and stromal cancer.* About 90% of ovarian cancers develop from epithelial—that is the lining membrane of the ovaries. Other cancers arise from germ or egg cells found in the ovaries as well as from stromal cells which make up the ovarian structure. Epithelial cancer can spread to the other ovary, pelvis and abdomen but do not invade deeper layers of tissue. Germ cell cancer affects the younger women and is not so common.

SYMPTOMS

Distension of abdomen, digestive troubles and gas. Sometimes fluid collects in the abdomen and there is abnormal vaginal bleeding. Frequent and urgent urination. Menstrual disorders and pain during intercourse.

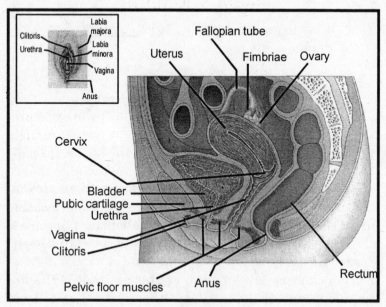

Female

CAUSES

Child birth, oral contraceptives, family history , breast cancer and colon cancer are usual causes of ovarian cancer.

DIAGNOSTIC TESTS

X-rays, ultrasound scan and blood tests are employed to detect its presence.

SURGERY

During the operation, one or both of the ovaries are removed. Often, the uterus and fallopian tubes are also removed partially to avoid the danger of the cancer spreading there or when the cancer has actually spread to them. *A pregnant women rarely develops ovarian cancer, if she does, the cancer remains in the ovary and the women carries the baby to a full term.* Taking out ovaries does not affect sexual activity and if only one ovary is removed, she still can have children.

DIET

A diet rich in fruits and vegetables can decrease the risk of ovarian cancer.

HOMOEOPATHIC TREATMENT

ALUMEN 30C : Cancer of the ovary with obstinate constipation.

BARYTA IODATA 3X : A remedy for cancerous tumors of the ovaries.

LACHESIS 200C : In the cancer of ovary, when there is induration and pain extending from left to the right ovary. Pains go on increasing until relieved by flow of blood from vagina. This condition happens again and again. Give this remedy one dose every 4th day. It acts on both the ovaries.

OOPHORINUM 3X   : Suffering following removal of the ovaries surgically.

Chapter-23

PANCREATIC CANCER

STRUCTURE

Pancreas is an elongated pinkish-yellowish gland lying directly behind the stomach and extends across the abdomen towards the back of the abdominal cavity. Its head is attached to the curve of the duodenum. Its body and tail stretch out to touch the spleen. It has two major functions, first to produce the insulin hormone which regulates blood sugar levels and secondly to produce digestive enzymes. Cells which produce digestive enzymes are clumped into groups called *'acini'* that lead into ducts through which the enzymes are delivered into the duodenum. The pancreatic duct eventually joins the bile duct through which bile is drained from the liver. Insulin converts carbohydrates or sugar to blood sugar. More than 90% of pancreatic cancer arise in the ductal cells which transport digestive enzymes to the duodenum. Often these cancers are surrounded by inflammed pancreatic tissue and cause pancreatitis. Tumors in the head of pancreas can obstruct the pancreatic and bile ducts causing jaundice. Cancer cells from these tumors often spread to the adjacent tissue, nearby lymph nodes and the liver.

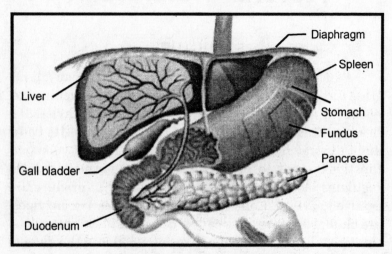

Location of the Pancreas

SYMPTOMS

1. A vague pain in the upper stomach.

2. Persistant backache.

3. Jaundice.

4. White stools and yellow urine.

5. Fatigue, trembling, chills, headache and anxious feeling.

CAUSES

Cigarette smoking, caffein consumption, eating diets high in fats from animal sources, certain chemicals found in coke and some industrial compounds are often linked to such cancers. *Diabetic women are at greater risk. Such cancers grow rapidly.*

DIAGNOSTIC TESTS

It is done by following methods:-

1. Ultrasound imaging.

2. Endoscopic Retrograde Cholangiopancreatography (ERCP). This method consists of passing a long, thin, flexible tube (endoscope) through the mouth into the stomach and duodenum and thereafter into the pancreatic duct. Pancreatic cells floating in the digestive fluids are removed for examination.

3. CAT Scan.

4. Biopsy.

SURGERY

The whole of the pancreas is removed and sometimes the head of panceas, the first portion of the small intestines, part of the stomach, the common bile duct and surrounding lymph nodes are all removed if the cancer has spread to these areas.

HOMOEOPATHIC TREATMENT

CALCAREA ARSENIC : Relieves burning pain of cancer in the pancreas.

IODINE 6X : Cancer of pancreas with rapid emaciation. The patient has canine hunger and eats lot of food but still loses flesh. He is always hungry because eating relieves his discomfort temporily. He feels worse in summer and warm room.

PHOSPHORUS 200C : Fatty degeneration of the pancreas. Oily-looking stools. Excessively bleeding cancer of the pancreas. A dose every seventh day.

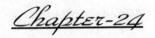

PENIS CANCER

STRUCTURE

The male organ of copulation and urination. It is a cylindrical pendulous organ suspended from the front and sides of the pubic arch.

SYMPTOMS

Penis cancer is generally found in men, past the middle age. The prepuce and glans are the parts most commonly affected. A small wart-like tumor first appears. It finally ulcerates and developes fungus growths and oozes fetid and bloody matter. As the disease advances, it extends to abdomen and later involves the inguinal and adjacent glands.

CAUSES

Exact cause is not known but it is believed that the syphilitic ulcer may develop into this kind of cancer.

HOMOEOPATHIC TREATMENT

AURUM METALLICUM 30C :   Hard lump on the middle of

the shaft of penis. A cartilaginous tumor.

PHYTOLACCA Q : When the cancer develops fungus growth and the discharge is fetid pus. The head of penis is swollen.

SCROPHULARIA Q : A large growth on the head of the penis involving most of its parts and the enlarged surrounding glands. Apply locally also.

STRYCHNINUM SULPHURICUM 30C : Cramp-like pains in the penis and surrounding areas with rigidity and twitching or jerking. Cold feeling.

Chapter-25

PROSTATE CANCER

STRUCTURE

Prostate gland is located below the bladder and in front of the rectum and is about the size of a walnut. It secretes a fluid which carries the sperms and forms a part of semen.

SYMPTOMS

1. Frequent, difficult or painful urination.

2. Dribbling of urine.

3. Blood or pus in the urine.

4. Pain in the lower back, pelvic area or upper thigh.

5. Painful ejaculation.

CAUSES

No definite cause of prostate cancer is known, but older people are more likely to develop such a cancer. Excessive use of aluminium in water or in foods is believed to be one cause.

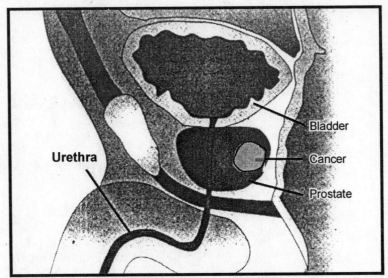

Cancer confined to the Prostate

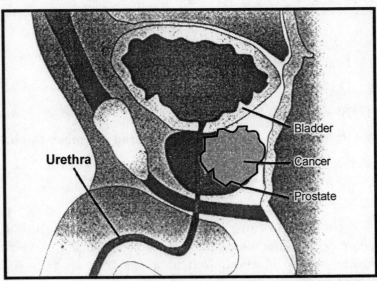

Locally advanced cancer

DIAGNOSTIC TESTS

1. Digital rectal examination.
2. PSA Blood test.
3. Transrectal ultrasound scan.
4. Biopsy.

TREATMENT

When prostate cancer is found in the prostate gland and has not spread further, it is removed surgically. Radiation, hormone treatment or a combination of these treatments are used to stop the growth of and destroy the cancer cells. By an operation, the cancerous prostate gland is removed, usually it is done through an incision in the lower abdomen. Such surgery is called radical retropubic prostatectomy. These procedures cause impotency in about 66% of cases, because the two nerves which carry signals to the penis to fill with blood allowing erections are injured or removed alongwith the cancerous prostate glands.

HOMOEOPATHIC TREATMENT

CADMIUM PHOSPHATE 30C : It is useful in the treatment of carcinoma of the prostate gland. Persistant vomiting is usually present.

CINNAMONUM Q : Cancer is painful and bleeding. The discharge is offensive.

CISTUS CANADENSIS 30C : Prostate cancer with fetid discharge. The patient is extremely sensative to cold and has a sensation of coldness in various parts.

CROTALUS HORRIDUS 30C : Cancer with bleeding of the prostate gland. It reduces pain of the cancer.

HOANG NAN Q	: A useful remedy for this disease. Start with 5 drops three times a day and gradually increase to 20 drops.
LYCOPODIUM 1M	: Cures prostate carcinoma. The patient is emaciated and feels very weak in the morning. Backache before urination and which disappears after it.
PROSTATE CANCER VACCINE	: Prostate cancer patients are being effectively treated by using vaccine prepared from their own cancer. It is prepared from the blood drawn from the cancer. Its use shrinks the cancer and puts on hold its growth.

NOTE:-

1. Eating tomatoes reduces the risk of cancer of prostate. Tomato contains Vitamins A, B-complex and C as well as iron and potassium. Red tomatoes contain lycopene which protects against variety of ailments. Lycopene is also found in watermelon and papaya.

2. Use of foods containing selenium also reduces the risk of prostate cancer. Selenium is found in minute quantity in meat, fish, whole grains, dairy products and vegetables grown in the selenium-rich soil.

Chapter-26

SCROTUM CANCER

STRUCTURE

The double pouch of the male, which contains testicles and part of the spermatic cord. It is formed by network of nonstriated muscular fibres and muscles.

SYMPTOMS

A small ulcer at the base of the scrotum becomes malignant and spreads rapidly to the testicles and adjacent parts. It discharges foul-smelling liquid.

SURGERY

Scrotectomy, that is excision of part of scrotum.

HOMOEOPATHIC TREATMENT

ARSENIC ALBUM 30C : Cancer is painful and burning. Pain and burning is relieved by hot water bath and warm applications. The pain is worse at the midnight.

AURUM METALLICUM 30C: The swelling of the cancer is hard

but tender. The pain is worse at night.

FULIGO LIGNI 3X
: A special remedy for treatment of cancer of scrotum. Epithelioma due to chronic irritation by coal soot, that is, chimney sweep cancer.

MAGNESIUM PHOSPHORICUM 6X
: Neuralgic pain in the cord relieved by light pressure and warmth.

PHYTOLACCA Q
: This should be painted on the cancer twice daily. If there is aching, soreness, restlessness and debility. Give five drops internally three times a day.

Chapter-27

SKIN CANCER AND MYELOMA

STRUCTURE

There are three kinds of the skin cancer—*Basal cell carcinoma, Squamous cell carcinoma and Myeloma,* and if detected early all of them are curable. About 80 % of the skin cancers are basal cell and squamous cell carcinomas.

SYMPTOMS

1. **Basal cell:** Painless smooth slowly growing lump usually on the face, ears or neck.

2. **Squamous cell:** Painless scaly reddish lump usually on the face, ears, neck, arms or hands.

3. **Myeloma:** Painless mole with irregular shape located anywhere on the body and which refuses to heal.

CAUSES

Fair skin with freckles having many moles. Red or blond hair and light-colored eyes. The risk of melonoma increases greatly after the age of 50 years. Exposure to

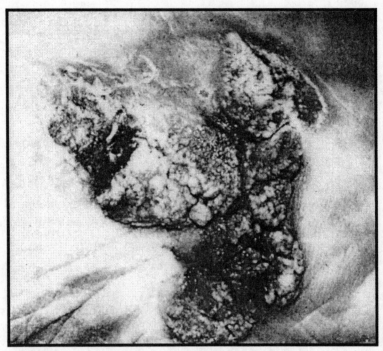
Squamous cell cancer

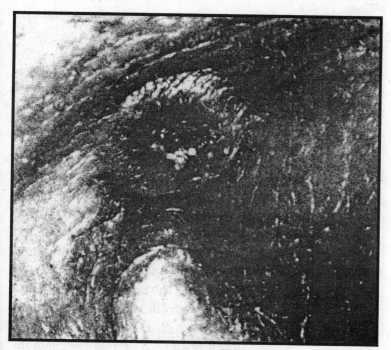

Basal cell cancer

ultra voilet rays, coal tar, creosote, arsenic compounds and family history are other causes.

DIAGNOSTIC TESTS

Microscopic examination of the suspected cells and biopsy.

SURGERY

It includes *cryosurgery* (tissue destruction by freezing), *Laser therapy* (destruction with laser rays) and *electrodesiccation* (tissue destruction by heat).

HOMOEOPATHIC TREATMENT

ARSENIC 3C-200 : Cancer arising from overgrowth of fibrous tissues or a cancer originating from the epidermis of the skin—may be hard or soft. Start the treatment with 3C potency and give it four times a day and go on selecting the potency which effects the most. If this remedy cannot cure, it will atleast reduce the pain and maintain or restore the general health.

CANNABIS SATIVA Q : Fatty acids found in hemp protect the skin against sun. 15 drops in half a cup of water is used for protection of the skin against the skin cancer due to the sun rays.

EUPHORBIUM 6C : Ulcerating carcinoma and epithelioma of the skin.

HYDRASTIS 30C	: Cancerous formation on the skin. Skin is ulcerated with smallpox like eruptions.
KALIUM ARSENIC 30C	: Skin cancer with no other visible symptoms except many small nodules under the sun.
LOBELIA ERINUS 30C	: Epithelioma, that is malignant tumor consisting principally of epithelial cells and originating from the epidermis of the skin or in a mucous membrane and developing rapidly. Dryness of the skin, nose and mucous membrane of the cheeks.
RADIUM BROM	: Cancer of skin with itching, burning and restlessness. Epithelioma.

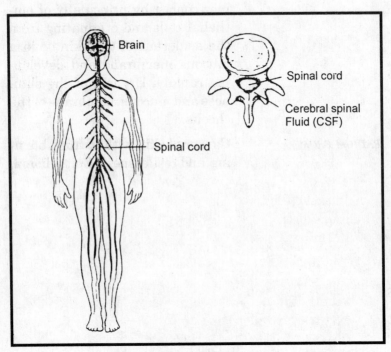

Location of Spinal cord
with the vertebra

Chapter-28

SPINAL CORD CANCER

STRUCTURE

Spinal cord is essentially an extension of the brain. It lies in the centre of the vertebrae known as backbone. It conducts signals along nerve fibres between the brain and other parts of the body. Bathing spinal cord is a watery solution called the Cerebro Spinal Fluild (CSF). Spinal cord is protected by a body shell and by three layers of membranes called the meninges.

SYMPTOMS

1. Headache is the most common symptom.
2. Vomiting with or without nausea.
3. Progressive muscular weakness and lack of coordination.
4. Trouble with balance.
5. Blurred or double vision.
6. Seizures.
7. Personality changes.
8. Memory Loss.

9. Numbness and weakness if the tumor has developed in the cone of the spinal cord.

CAUSES

There is no known cause of primary tumor of the spinal cord. Evidence, however, exists indicating that persons working in the petrochemical industry may have a higher risk of developing such tumors. Many types of tumors that start in the brain also start in the spinal cord.

DIAGNOSTIC TESTS

1. X-Rays.

2. Computerized Axial Tomography (CAT) Scan.

3. Electroencephalogram (EEG).

4. Nuclear Magnatic Resonance Imaging (MRI).

5. Angiogram.

6. Biopsy.

SURGERY

Surgery can only be performed in the operable locations by sophisticated surgical instruments such as operating microscope.

HOMOEOPATHIC TREATMENT

BACILLINUM 200C	: A weekly dose before and after the start of the treatment.
CALCAREA SULPHURICUM 6X	: Tumor becomes ulcerative and discharges pus of yellow colour.
STRYCHNIA PHOSPHORICUM 3X	: Aching and burning of the spine. Mid-dorsal region tender to pres-

sure. The patient is declined to use the brain. Lack of control of muscles and their coordination. Muscular weakness.

NOTE : If the tumor is too large due to the fluid contained in it, put a bandage or any other support to avoid its hanging down and putting weight on the spine. It is better to refer the case to a competent surgeon if tumor resists the treatment.

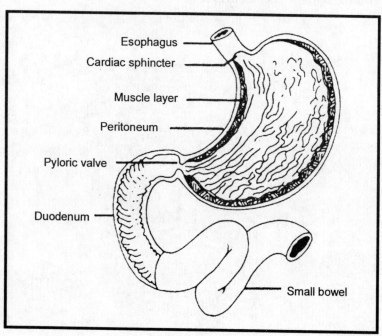

Stomach

Chapter-29

STOMACH CANCER

STRUCTURE

The human stomach is a muscular, elastic, pear-shaped bag that lies in the abdominal cavity and conveys food from the esophagus to the intestines. As a part of the digestive tract, the stomach is capable of enormous alterations in both size and shape, depending upon the food contained in it. In humans, it is about 12 inches in length and about 6 inches in the diameter at its widest point.An adult stomach can hold one litre of food on a average. It is made up of three layers. The outer layer is fibrous, the middle layer is of muscle and the innermost layer which is made up of some 35000 glands. The innermost layer appears like a honeycomb when the stomach is empty. These glands secrete gastric acid and gastric juices which reduce the food to a semi-liquid state. A few foods including simple sugars and alcohol can actually be absorbed into the body directly through the stomach wall. Then most of the food passes into the intestines where absorption takes place. Scirrhus is the most common form of the disease but sometimes it take the form of epithelioma. Cancer of the stomach is like all other cancers in general. In almost all cases, it begins in the innermost (glandular) layer and on growing, it invades the adjacent layer and extends. After many months and sometimes many years, some of the cancerous cells may break up from the primary tumor and spread through the bloodstream or lymphatic system to the liver and lungs. The adjacent organs like pancreas and the spleen may be infected directly from the walls of the stomach. It is called the advanced cancer of the stomach. The favourite seat of cancer is pylorus and the duodenum.

SYMPTOMS

1. Vague digestive discomfort.

2. Mild lancinating and burning pain in the abdomen which may extend to the back of the spine.

3. Slight but persistent nausea and heartburn and vomiting after eating.

4. Blood in the stools.

5. Extreme fatigue.

6. Rapid weight loss.

7. Tenderness of the stomach region, the patient cannot bear the touch of hand over his stomach.

CAUSES

Stomach cancer generally attacks people:-

1. Who have undergone surgery of the stomach.

2. Who eat diets higher in starch and lower in fibre i.e. fresh fruits and vegetables.

3. Who eat preserved and smoked food.

4. Who have had pernicious anemia or who suffer from achlorhydria (absence of hydrochloric acid in the gastric

secretions) or who are suffering from Helicobacter pylori infection of the stomach.

5. Eating too much and too fast.

DIAGNOSTIC TESTS

It is done by gastroscopy, X-ray examination and biopsy.

SURGERY

In order to remove the tumor, a part or the entire stomach may have to be removed. Sometimes affected spleen and pancreas are also removed. Treatment with chemotherapy may also occur.

DIET

Even if the entire stomach is removed, the post operative difficulties in digestion can usually be prevented by eating simple food in small quantity several times a day. Diets low in carbohydrates and high in proteins and fats are useful. Vegetables, like tomatoes, carrots and turnips when well cooked are all good. Tea, coffee and alcohol should not be taken.

HOMOEOPATHIC TREATMENT

ACETIC ACIDUM 1X-30 : Cancer of stomach, voilent burning pains in the stomach and chest followed by coldness of the skin and cold perspiration on the forehead. Anemia. Bleeding from bowels. Its use dissolves the cancer cells in the stomach. Epithelial cancer and cancer of layers lining the cavities of the alimentary canal.

ARSENIC ALBUM 30C	: Vomiting of blood, bile, green mucus or brown black mixed with blood. Great thirst—drinks often but little at a time. Everything swallowed seems to lodge in the esophagus and does not move down. Fixed burning pain in the stomach.
BELLIS PERENNIS 30C	: Cancer of stomach with burning pain in the esophagus.
BISMUTHUM 30C	: Very easy vomiting of clear water or enormous quantities of food which appears to have laid in the stomach for days.
CADMIUM SULPHURICUM 30 C	: Very slowly developing cancer of the stomach with persistant vomiting.
CARBO VEGETABILIS 30C	: There is excessive flatulence in the stomach and there are loud eructations from the mouth. The stomach feels full and tense from large quantities of gas which produces great pain that is rendered more intense by lying down.
CAUSTICUM 30C	: The flesh over the stomach is very tender and the patient does not bear even touch of clothing to it. Lightest food or lightest of pressure over the stomach causes lancinating pains.
COLOCYNTH 30C	: This remedy is indicated in sharp lancinating pains shooting down the bowels in case of cancer at the

pyloric orifice of the stomach.

CONDURANGO 30C : Cancer of stomach accompanied in most cases with painful cracks in the corners of the mouth. Vomiting of food and constant cramping and burning pain behind sternum. Relieves cancer pains. Even a touch on stomach causes pain.

CROTALUS HORRIDUS 30C: Cancer of stomach with constant nausea and vomiting of bloody, slimy mucus. Cannot tolerate any clothing around the epigastrium.

DIOSCOREA : Stomach seems full of gas with griping pains.

EUCALYPTUS GLOB Q : In case of cancer of stomach when there is vomiting of blood mixed with sour fluid and fetid smell. Give 25 drops twice daily.

GERANIUM MACULATUM : Hemorrhage from stomach due to a cancer in it. Give 25 drops every hour till the bleeding stops.

GRAPHITIS 200C : One dose a week for cancer of pylorus and duodenum.

HYDRASTIS : Ulcers and cancer of the stomach with pulsation in the epigastrium and gastritis. Flatulence and distress in the bowels after meals.

IODIUM 1X : In cancer of stomach when patient has ravenous hunger but loses flesh all the time. Hunger is relieved by eating for the time being, when he feels hungry again.

KREOSOTUM 30C	: Bad smelling vomiting after eating. Burning pain in the stomach.
LOBELIA ERINUS 30C	: Cancer of the walls of peritonium of stomach, developing rapidly. Cork screw like pains in the abdomen.
NUX VOMICA 200C	: Vomiting of sour fluid. A dose daily.
ORNITHOGALUM Q	: Painful sinking across epigastrium and belching of offensive gas. Loss of weight and flesh. Vomiting of coffee ground looking matter sometimes accompanied with blood. Cancer anywhere in the intestinal tract, especially in the lower part of the stomach before start of the intestines. Three doses per day for four days and then await results before repeating.
PHOSPHORUS 30C	: Vomiting of food and water after it gets warm in the stomach. Difficulty in swallowing of food. Stomach pain is relieved by cold drinks and ice.
TUBERCULINUM 1000C	: Carcinoma of the stomach. The patient is always hungry and tired. Use it when well-selected remedies fail to improve and there is rapid emaciation. *Should not be prescribed for patients having heart, skin and intestinal affections.* Do not repeat it before 15 days of the first dose and watch the results.

Chapter-30

TESTICULAR CANCER

STRUCTURE

The testes are contained in the scrotum, a pouch of skin at the base of the penis. Surrounding the testes is a thin membrane called a tunic. Running along the near of the scrotum are the epididymides, long coiled ducts in which the sperms mature and are stored until they migrate into the ductus deferenes on their way to the tip of the penis. The spermatic cord also runs through the scrotum and consists of arteries, veins and nerves. Compared to other cancers of the male organs, cancer of testicles is rare but it is most common type seen in men aged 29-35 years.

SYMPTOMS

1. A lump in either testicles.
2. Any engorgement of the testicles.
3. Feeling of heaviness in the scrotum.
4. A dull ache in the lower abdomen or groin.
5. Blood in the urine.
6. Engorgement and tenderness of the breasts.

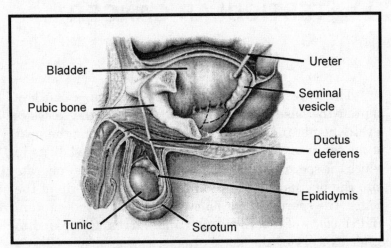

Testicle

CAUSES

Cryptochidism, that is, failure of testicles to descend into the scrotum is regarded as one of the causes. Some infants are born with this condition. Injury to the testicles can also cause this cancer. A child born of a mother who took estrogen hormones during pregnancy or before it can have it. This type of cancer is extremely rare in blacks.

DIAGNOSTIC TESTS

Because testicular cancer occurs in an external organ, it can be detected by finding a lump by self examination. Other signs include dull pain in the groin, abdomen or flank, enlargement of male breasts like females and lumps in the neck. CAT Scan, Lymphangiography, Biopsy and Blood tests can also detect such cancers.

SURGERY

Usually testicular cancer develops in one testicle only and when the cancerous testicle is removed, the other testicle takes up its functions and produces enough sperms to make up the loss of one testicle. Hence it does not affect sterility or sexuality.

DIET

The patient can eat anything, better vegetarian, whatever suits him.

HOMOEOPATHIC TREATMENT

ARSENIC ALBUM 1M   : A carcinoma originating from the epidermis of the skin of the scrotum.

AURUM METALLICUM 30C:	Cancer of the testes due to accumulation of serous fluid.
CADMIUM PHOSPHORICUM 30C	: Cancer of the testicles when there is extreme prostration and vomiting.
CONIUM 1M	: Cancer of testicles which become hard and enlarged. Breasts look like that of a woman. Give a dose fortnightly for a long time.
FULIGO LIGNI 3X	: Cancer of scrotum. Epitheloma due to chronic irritation by coal soot. (Chimney Sweep Cancer).
RHODODENDRON 30C	: Cancer of the left testicle. The testicle is drawn up, swollen and painful.
SPONGIA 2X	: Cancer of testicles with swelling of the testicles. Swelling spreads to the spermatic cord. Painful. Pain is worse while ascending and before midnight.

Chapter-31

THROAT CANCER

STRUCTURE

Throat consists of the cavity from the arch of the palate to the glottis and the opening of the oesophagus in the anterior portion of the neck. It contains pharynx and the fauces.

SYMPTOMS

A sharp shooting pain in the throat and difficulty in swallowing. The throat appears blocked. The breath is foul. Tongue is coated dirty yellow.

HOMOEOPATHIC TREATMENT

NYMPHAEA ODORATA Q : 10 drops of the tincture in half a cup of water three times a day can cure cancer of throat. It is an excellent remedy where there is also backache and morning diarrhoea.

PHYTOLACCA DECANDRA Q : This is a *leading remedy in the cancer of throat.* Give 5 drops in little water thrice daily. This should also be used for gurgling.

THUJA 200C : Spongy tumor of throat without ulceration. This can be considered as rival to phytolacca in such cases.

Chapter-32

THYROID CANCER

STRUCTURE

The thyroid gland is yellowish-red mass of butterfly shaped grandular tissue. It is located at the base of the neck on both sides of the lower part of the larynx and upper part of trachea. Histologically it consists of a large number of closed vessels called follicles which contain a homogenous substance called colloid. Colloid contains various active substances such as thyroxine and tri-iodo-thyronine. These have far reaching effects on the body. These hormones aid the cells to burn oxygen and break down glucose to produce energy. Cancer of thyroid is a less frequently occuring form of cancer.

SYMPTOMS

Cancer of thyroid gland develops slowly and remains localised. This usually appears as nodules or lumps in the neck of tissue growing on or inside of the gland. Most lumps in the neck are caused by goitres. There are four types of thyroid cancer—*papillary, follicular, medullary* and *anaplastic. Papillary thyroid tumor* occur more commonly. It develops on one or both sides of the gland and

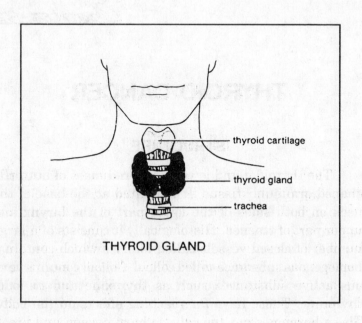

thyroid cartilage

thyroid gland

trachea

THYROID GLAND

remains confined for several years. *Follicular tumors* grow only on one side of the gland. *Anaplastic tumors,* though extremely rare, develop quickly and spread rapidly to other parts of the body. *Medullary carcinomas* of the thyroid are also uncommon but are sometimes hereditary.́

CAUSES

Evidence suggests that external radiation to the neck and head areas may cause thyroid cancer in some people. It can take 20-40 years or longer for the cancer to appear in such cases.

DIAGNOSTIC TESTS

1. Thyroid scan is done after 24-48 hours after taking of very minute amounts of radioactive substance called isotope given by mouth or by injection.

2. Ultrasound imaging.

3. Fine needle biopsy.

SURGERY

During surgery either a part of or the entire thyroid is removed. The procedure is called *thyroidectomy.* When whole of the thyroid is removed, thyroid pills are to be taken for life time. Frequently, radioactive iodine is used to treat this type of cancer. This is administered almost invariably after primary surgery for metastasis.

HOMOEOPATHIC TREATMENT

IODIUM 6X   : Thyroid gland is enlarged with cancerous developments. Larynx feels constricted. Swollen lymphatic nodes in the armpits. Great debility and rapid emaciation but with very good appitite.

LOBELIA ERINUS 30C : Colloidal cancer of the thyroid with extremely rapid development extending to stomach and abdomen. Cork-screw like pains are felt in the stomach. The glue like secretion of thyroid gland becomes defective.

Chapter-33

TONGUE CANCER

STRUCTURE

A freely movable muscular organ lying partly in the floor of the mouth and partly on the pharynx. Its function is manipulation of food in mastication and deglutition, speech articulation and taste. Its surface is covered with mucous membrane.

SYMPTOMS

A fungus-like growth on the side or underneath the tongue. The tongue is hard and there may be fissures on the tongue. The pains are like those produced by pricking of a needle and extend to the throat and the head. The cancer bleeds easily.

CAUSES

Causes are obscure.

HOMOEOPATHIC TREATMENT

CHROMICUM ACID 3X   : Epithelioma of tongue with foul smelling breath.

CROTALUS HORRIDUS 6C :	Cancer of the tongue with hemorrhage of dark blood that forms no clot.
GALIUM APARINE Q :	It is a useful remedy for treatment of the cancerous ulcers and nodulated tumors of the tongue. It favors healthy granulations on the ulcerated surfaces. Use half a dram dose in a cup of water three times a day.
KALIUM CYANATUM 3X :	In the last stages of cancer of tongue when the pain is very severe. The patient cannot eat a full meal.
LEMON JUICE :	Often effective for pains of the cancer of tongue—a tablespoonful every three hours. It can also be used as mouth wash—one dram to 8 ounces of water.
SEMPERVIVUM TECTORUM 3X :	Hard cancer of the tongue when the side of the tongue is ulcerated and is very sore and painful. The whole mouth seems to be tender and sensative. Tongue is ulcerated and bleeds easily especially at night. Dose 10 drops mixed with an ounce of water three times a day.
VIBURNUM PRUNIFOLIUM :	Cancer of the tongue.

Chapter-34

UTERINE CANCER

STRUCTURE

Uterus is a muscular, hollow, pear-shaped structure and is partly covered by the peritonium and the cavity is covered by mucous membrane called endometrium. This female organ contains and nourishes the embryo and fetus from the time the fertilized egg is implanted in it to the time of birth of the fetus. There are two different types of uterine cancer. One is the cancer of cervix or cervical cancer, the other is cancer of endometrium or endometrial cancer. Both, otherwise, have characteristics of cancers in general. Cervical cancer is mostly a disease of young women while endometrial cancer mostly affects older women. In most cases of cervical cancer, the cells covering the cervix undergo mild to severe changes for some years before becoming cancerous which are then called *dysplasia*. Similarly the cells of lining of the uterus (endometrial tissue) after undergoing changes becomes cancerous which are then called *hyperplasia*. Upto 90 % of cervical cancers are of squamous cell type, the rest are adenosquamous carcinoma. It is not necessary that the pre-cancerous conditions must become cancerous. If the cancers are not treated, the cancerous cells can penetrate the deeper layer of the uterus and spread to the neighbouring organs like lymph nodes, vagina, bladder and rectum. They can also spread to lungs.

SYMPTOMS

The usual symptoms are heavy menstruation lasting longer with excruciating pains.

CAUSES

Studies have shown that those who begin their sex lives before the age of 17 years and have many partners, are very much susceptible to cervical cancer. Cervix is the neck of the womb or uterus. Women between the age of 50-74 years who are obese or continue to menstruate after 50 years of age or show signs of hypertension, or are sterile can suffer from endometrial cancer. Endometrium is the lining of the uterus. It rarely occurs before menopause.

DIAGNOSTIC TESTS

Pap test is performed to detect cervical cancer. A thin wooden spatula which is smaller than the tongue depressor is inserted into the cervix through the vagina and is rotated to scrape the cells. These are tested in a laboratory to determine whether these are cancerous or otherwise. Pap test should be done every year for the first three years after a women becomes sexually active. A visual examination can be made by the aid of calposcope by which little portions of the tissue are taken to perform biopsy.

SURGERY

Cryosurgery or laser therapy is used to destroy abnormal areas of the cervix. In more serious cases, the cervix, uterus, tubes and lymph nodes of the areas are removed. Ovaries may or may not be removed. When the cancer has spread to other areas of the body, chemotherapy (treatment with anti-cancer drugs) is prescribed. In most of the cases, surgeons suggest *hysterectomy* (removal of uterus). This procedure ends fertility and produces menopause. Most women therefore, prefer alternate treatment which is called *Uterine Fibroid Embolization (UFE)*. This procedure involves an incision of the size of a pencil tip made into groin. From it a catheter is guided through an artery to the uterus. Small plastic particles are injected into the vessels supplying blood to the fibroid and block the vessels cutting off blood supply to the fibroid causing it to shrink and die eventually. This procedure does not interfere with the normal functions of the female reproductive system like menstruation and fertility.

HOMOEOPATHIC TREATMENT

APIS MELLIFICA : Ovarian cancer with great tenderness over the region of uterus and stinging pains. Sensative to touch.

AURUM ARSENICUM 30C : Uterine cancer with increased sexual desire.

AURUM IODATUM 3X : Inoperable fibroma or myoma of uterus with very offensive bloody discharge.

AURUM MURIATICUM NATRONATUM 3X : A powerful remedy for cure of cancer of the uterus. Cancer fills up the whole uterus and whole pelvis. The use of this remedy reduces the size of cancer and finally cures it.

CADMIUM
SULPHURICUM CM
: After radiotherapy , chemotherapy and other alternative treatments, if the cancer still persist—a dose be given every fortnight for a sufficient long time to cure the disease.

CALCAREA IODIUM 3X
: A good remedy in fibroid tumors of the uterus when the growth is tender with sharp darting pains.

CARBO VEGETABILIS. 30C: This remedy effects cancerous discharges and revives the dormant energies of the system.

CARCINOSIN 200C
: Carcinoma of uterus. A state of ill health and wasting. Loss of weight. Relieves bleeding and pain.

CHROMIUM
SULPHATE 3X
: Fibroid tumor of the uterus with bloody foul smelling discharge from vagina.

FICUS INDICA Q
: Hemorrhage from uterus due to a cancer in it.

FRAXINUS AMERICANA Q: 10-15 drops a dose thrice daily is helpful for treatment of fibroma of uterus.

HELONIAS 6X
: Pain and weight in the back. Burning sensation inside the uterus and this feeling extends to the legs. Menses too profuse and too frequent. Sensation of weakness, dragging and weight in the sacrum

and pelvis with prostration. Prolapse of womb.

HYDRASTIS Q : This remedy is undoubtedly useful when the cancerous growth involves the glands of the uterus. It can be used internally as well as externally. There can be acrid and corroding shreddy and tenacious menorrhagia and profuse leucorrhea.

HYDROCOTYLE Q : Uterine cancer pains are relieved by use of this remedy.

KREOSOTUM 6X : There is great burning in the pelvis like red hot coals. The discharge from uterus is foul and clotty.

LACHESIS 200C : If there is relief from the intense pain after bleeding of dark composed blood.

LAPIS ALBUS 6X : Carcinoma or fibroid tumor with intense burning pains and profuse foul smelling, black colored bleeding.

MUREX PURPUREA 6X : There is great depression. Pain in the uterus is as if cut by a knife, etc. It is lancinating and throbbing. The acrid discharge from uterus irritates the pudenda and thighs causing them to swell. Fainting " all gone" feeling in the stomach.

NATRIUM ACETICUM 6C : Cancer of uterus with pains and bleeding and foul breathing.

PHYTOLACCA Q	: 5 drops in little water thrice daily has a positive effect in fibroid tumors and cancers of the uterus.
PSORALEA 30C	: Uterine cancer accompanied by fetid leucorrhea and pruritus. Pain of the cancer.
PULSATILLA 30C	: Fibroid tumor near the fundus.
SALIDAGO VIGRA 30C	: Fibroid tumor of the uterus. There is obstruction to the flow of urine. Sometimes use of this remedy makes the employment of catheter unnecessary. Backache.
SEMPERVIVUM TECTORIUM 2X	: Vagina becomes very irritable and dry due to a cancer of uterus.
THLASPI BURSA Q	: Cancer or fibroma of uterus with cramps. Severe pain in the womb on rising. Hemorrhage with voilent uterine colic.
THUJA 200C	: Cauliflower type of cancer of uterus and fungus growth.
USTILAGO MAYDIS Q	: Fibroid tumor of uterus with profuse menstruation. Burning sensation in the uterus. Oozing of dark, clotted and stingy blood from vagina.

Chapter-35

CANCER OF VAGINA

STRUCTURE

A tube formed by muscles and mucous membranes which acts as a passage between the uterus and the vaginal orifice. Its function is to serve as passage for introduction of the penis and reception of semen. It serves as a gate for discharge of menstrual flow and also as a birth canal.

SYMPTOMS

A very painful tumor or an open ulcer at the lower end of the vagina or near the opening of urethra or on the labia. The pains come and go and extend to the thighs and knees. The pain is very extreme during urination. This generally occurs during or after menopausal periods.

SURGERY

Vaginectomy i.e. excision of the vagina or a part of it.

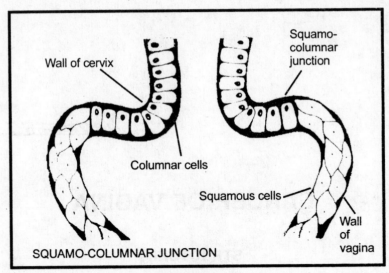

Cervical cancer

HOMOEOPATHIC TREATMENT

KREOSOTUM 30C : Cancer of vagina with burning pain.

SILICEA 6X : Three grains a dose three times a day.

THUJA 200C : One dose every four days. Externally *Thuja Q* should be painted on the cancer three times a day.

Chapter-36

CANCER OF VULVA

STRUCTURE

It is a portion of the female genitalia and consists of clitoris and labiae i.e. the labia majora and labia minora.

SYMPTOMS

Diffuse or focal translucent thickening of vulva that afterwards gives rise to carcinoma.

SURGERY

Surgical operation is called 'vulvectomy'. The surgeon removes the whole vulva. This includes the inner and outer lips, the clitoris and often the lymph nodes. The vagina, uterus and ovaries remain intact. After the operation, women may have problems reaching orgasm because clitoris is an important part in women's sexual pleasure.

HOMOEOPATHIC TREATMENT

EUPIONUM 3C
: Severe backache extending to pelvis and sacrum. Sore pain between the labiae during urination. Labiae swollen. Gushing leucorrhea.

SANGUINARIA 30C
: Cancer of labia with burning sensation like from hot water. Fetid corrosive leucorrhea.

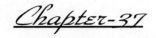

Chapter-37

FIVE STEPS TO PREVENT CANCERS

1. Avoid smoking—both direct and indirect.

2. Eat a variety of low fat, high fibre foods. Maintain a healthy body weight and do not take alcohol.

3. Protect from Sun rays.

4. Regularly have Pap tests, mammograms and breast examination.

5. Notice any change in health on discovery of a lump or a mole that has changed, or a sore that refuses to heal.

Chapter-38

DIET AND NUTRITION

After prescription for treatment, a question is often asked by a patient "Doctor, what should I eat". The food eaten gives strength, energy and stamina. A variety of foods stuff containing vitamins, minerals and proteins should be chosen during treatment of a cancer. Protein is important because it helps body to repair the tissues damaged due to a cancer. Fish, poultry and eggs provide many vitamins and minerals. Better vegetarian sources of proteins are beans, peas, lentils and nuts. Foods which supply fibres and important vitamins are fresh or cooked vegetables, fruits, salads and juices. Minerals and carbo-hydrates are provided by corn, wheat, rice, oats, whole-grain breads, buns and muffins. Milk also supplies a number of vitamins, minerals and proteins.

Studies have shown that cancer is more prevalent in the civilized and industrialized world than in the so called "Third World Countries" and India. The exact causes there of are not yet known but this has been associated with the intake of foods. Tea and coffee is weakens the nervous system and the coats of the stomach. In all countries where in take of tea and coffee excess, cancer cases are on increase. Meat eating is considered to be another cause of cancer .In countries where diet is almost entirely vegetarian, there are very few cases of cancer. Alcoholics suffer more from this disease than non-alcoholics. Smoking cigarrettes is the cause of lip, throat and lung cancer.

Most important measure to avoid the risk of cancer is living a simple life, eating simple vegetarian food, avoid alcohol drinking and smoking.

Chapter-39

TUMORS

Normal cells reproduce themselves throughout life but in an orderly and controlled manner. In the course normal growth, worn out tissues are replaced and wounds heal. When cells grow out of control and form a mass, the mass is called tumor. Some tumors grow and enlarge only at the site where they began and these are benign tumors. Other tumors not only enlarge locally but have the potential to invade and destroy the normal tissues around and to spread to the distant parts of the body. Such tumors are called malignant or cancer. Distant spread of a cancer occurs when malignant cells detach themselves from the original (primary) tumor, are carried to other parts of the body through blood or lymphatic vessels and establish themselves at the new site as a cancer. A tumor that has spread in this way is said to have metastasized and the secondary tumor or (tumors) is called metastasis. However, not all the localised growths are benign and not all the growths occuring at different sites are malignant. Genes are the blueprints that tell a cell when to divide and when to die. Often when a gene turns bad, it triggers uncontrolled growth; but genes called tumour suppressors step in to stop it. It is when these tumor suppressors also turn bad, that the tumors develop.

HOMOEOPATHIC MEDICINES USED FOR TREATMENT OF TUMORS

ALUMEN 200 : Tumor of ovaries with chronic constipation.

ARSENIC : For malignant tumors originating in the epidermis of skin, a carcinoma.

ASTERIAS RUBENS : Tumor of breasts. Acts on both breasts but better on left.

AURUM : Tumor of bones find this remedy useful when there are nightly bone pains.

AURUM MURIATICUM : A very good remedy for the uterine tumors.

AURUM ARSENICUM NATRONATUM 3X : Uterine cancer. Sexual desire increased. Inflammation of ovaries. Menses too copious, too frequent or absent.

BELLADONNA : Painful tumors of the breasts.

BUFO RANA : It is palliative in cancer of breasts.

CALCAREA

CARBONICA 200 : Brain tumor. Headache and vertigo on turning the head. Icy coldness of the head. May be used in fat patients. Pedunculated fibroid tumors with roots; and *Calc-p.* for fibroid tumors without roots, other indications of remedies must agree.

CALCAREA FLUORICA 200 : Hard tumor of abdomen, scalp and left breast.

CALCAREA IODIDE	: Uterine fibroids.
CALCAREA PHOSPHORICA 200	: May be used in thin persons. Brain tumor.
CHIMAPHILA Q	: Women with very large breasts and painful tumor of mammae, not ulcerated and with abundant milk.
COLOCYNTHIS	: Cystic tumors of the ovary.
CONDURANGO Q	: Hard tumor of the left breast.
CONIINUM	: Painful and hard tumor or cancer of either breast or both and that of uterus and stomach especially if the trouble started by injury to these parts.
CONIUM KALI CARB	: Tumors. Select the remedy according to the symptoms of the medicines.
EUCALYPTUS	: Use externally and internally in vascular tumors of female urethra.
FRAXINUS AMERICANA	: Fibroid tumors of the uterus with bearing down sensations. Dysmenorrhea.
HECLA LAVA	: A general remedy for tumors anywhere.
HYDRASTIS	: Tumors of breast hard and painful. Nipple retracted. Menorrhagia.
HYPERICUM	: Slow-developing tumors especially on the passage of nerves.
KALIUM CARBONICUM	: Cancer of womb with severe itching and cutting pains from hip to knee.

KALIUM IODICUM CM	: Womb packed with tumors. Patient is tired with numbness of legs. It causes disappearance of tumors and nodules of long standing.
KALIUM PHOSPHORICUM	: Remember it in the treatment of suspected malignant tumors.
KREOSOTE	: Cancer of uterus with very fetid oozing of blood. Epithelmic tumor of the lower lip with dry cracked skin.
LACHESIS 200	: Tumor or cancer of the left ovary or both ovaries. Pain in uterine region increases before menses and is relieved during menses.
LAPIS ALBUS	: Fibroid tumor or cancer of uterus with burning pains and debilitating bleeding.
MERCURIUS IODATUS FLAVUS	: Mammary tumors with warm perspiration.
NITRICUM ACIDUM 200	: Cystic tumor in the region of the ear lobes.
PALLADIUM	: Tumor of ovaries.
PHYTOLACCA	: Mammary tumors with enlarged axillary glands.
PULSATILLA 1M	: A dependable remedy for uterine fibroid tumors situated near fundus. A dose fortnightly.
SELENIUM	: Tumor of right breast.
SOLIDAGO VIGRA Q	: Uterine fibroid tumors pressing down on the bladder causing dif-

ficulties in passing urine.

STAPHYSAGRIA : Sebaceous tumors of the eyes. Tumor of the eyes containing oily, fatty matter.

TEUCRIUM CM : Polypus in vagina.

THIOSINAMINUM 2X : It is a great remedy for dissolving tumor. Use with indicated remedy.

THLASPI Q : Cancer or fibroid of uterus accompanied with hemorrhage and cramps and clots and aching in the back.

THUJA 200 : Brain tumors with migraine headache. Flatulence. Constipation. The patient is emotional and sentimental. Spongy tumors of the abdomen. Tumors of eyelids. Polypus of cervix of uterus. Irregular menses.

THYROIDINUM 2X : Fibroid tumor of breasts and uterus.

TRILLIUM : Very useful for hemorrhage from fibroids.

TUBERCULINUM 200 : A dose of this remedy should be given at the commencement of all sort of tumors.Specially for benign mammary tumors.

Chapter-40

CANCER PAINS

The following remedies reduce the pains or abolish them when indicated:-

ACIDUM PHOSPHORICUM IX	: It is useful in relieving pain of cancer, mental and physical debility.
APIS MELLIFICA 30C	: Stinging pains with swellings and extremely sensitive to touch. Specially useful in ovarian tumors when the heat is not tolerated.
ANTHRACINUM 3X	: Pains in the spleen with burning and its swelling.
ASTERIAS RUBENS 3C	: Lancinating pains in the cancer of breasts. Left breast feels pulled inward. Pain under sternum.
BRYONIA 30C	: Stitching, tearing and burning pains worse by motion and better by rest. Especially indicated when ovaries are affected.
CALCAREA ARSENICUM 3X	: Pains in liver and spleen worse from slightest exertion.

CALENDULA Q	: A powerful remedy used on the external cancers and makes the cancer to discharge the deseased matter. It reduces the burning and irritation and heals the wound. It is applied spread on lint or muslin cloth.
CARCINOSIN 200C	: This nosode is made of fluid drawn out of breast cancer. It is useful for great pain of the breast cancer which is hard. It is also useful for pains of uterus due to a cancer. It greatly relieves such pains.
CINNAMOMUM Q	: Pains in the uterine cancer accompanied by bleeding with offensive odor. Oil of cinnamomum in watery solution is a best disinfectant of external cancers when the skin is intact. It reduces the cancer pains and offensive odor of the cancer. Four drops in 2 litres of water can be used as a douche as a germicide and disinfectant in case of cancer of uterus, etc.
CONDURANGO Q	: Relieves pain of cancer of the stomach.
CONIUM 200C	: Lancinating pain of cancer of breasts and ovaries worse by mental exertion and lying down better from letting limbs hang down and motion.
ECHINACEA Q	: It has no curative effect in cases of cancers but its use eases the

pain in the last stages of a cancer. Locally it is used as cleansing and antiseptic wash of the cancerous parts. It has antibiotic and anti-fungal properties.

EUPHORBIUM 30C : It is a palliative for burning pains of cancer of bones or skin and pe-riodical cramps.

HYDRASTIS 30C : Pain in the lymphoma of neck, can-cer of throat, stomach, uterus, ure-thra and skin before ulceration.

IODIUM Q : Tincture iodine is used locally in cases of external cancers. It is very powerful, harmless, and easily managed microbicide. It keeps the cancerous wounds clean and dis-infected.

LEMON JUICE : A tablespoon full of lemon juice taken every three hours relieves cancer pains specially that of can-cer of tongue.

MAGNESIUM PHOSPHORICUM 12X : Neuralgic pains which are relieved by warmth, pressure and friction.

MAGNESIUM SULPHURICUM (Epson Salt) : For local use pure salt is mixed with water in the ratio 1 : 4. It relieves inflammation and itching of the cancerous parts.

MORPHINUM 6X : Bursting pains of cancer of the bladder.

OVA TOSTA 3X : Pains of ovaries due to a cancer. General remedy for cancer pains when backache is present.

PHYTOLACCA Q	: Mother tincture is applied externally on the breast with cancer to reduce swelling and inflammation.
SUNFLOWER OIL	: It is used externally to reduce soreness and as a healing agent of cancerous wounds.

Chapter-41

SEXUALITY AND CANCER

It is normal for people with cancer to have periods of disinterest in sex and loss of its desire because of the stress and concern about their health. Cancers are mostly detected after the age of 50 years and many people believe that sex is only for people younger than this age and hence they lose their desire for sex. These beliefs are largely myths. Men and women remain sexually active until the end of their life. Sexuality is a need for closeness, touch, playfulness, caring and pleasure. Even when sex become impractical due to the removal of cancerous genital parts, physical expression of caring remains an important way of sharing closeness. Cuddling can give enough pleasure. If the areas of genitals most sensitive to touch have undergone changes due to the operation for cancer, the favourite position for intercourse may have to be changed. Almost all people who could reach orgasm before cancer treatment can reach it after or during the treatment. A position should be found for touching and intercourse that puts as little pressure as possible on the painful areas of the body. In the society, the most favourite and common way to have intercourse is the man lying on the top of the women. During and after the surgical

Positions to help in resuming intercourse
after Cancer treament

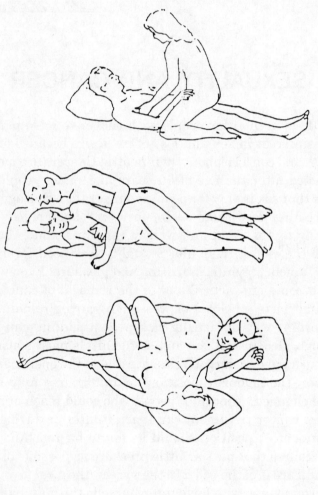

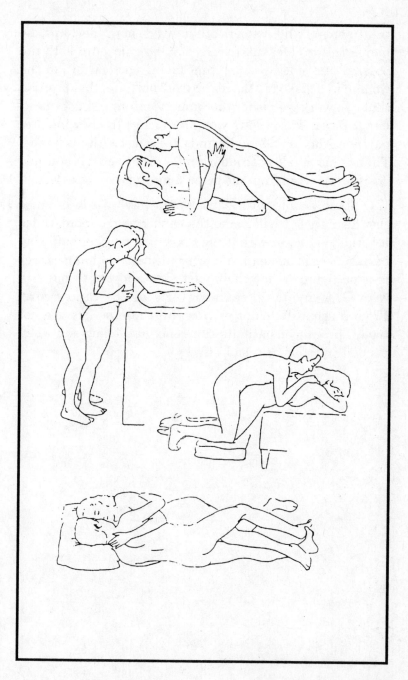

treatment of the cancer, other ways may, perhaps, be more comfortable. Intercourse can be enjoyed if both the partners lie side by side either facing each other , or the woman's back next to the man's front side. Another position that can work well is for the women is to sit or kneel aside her partner. This allows woman to move freely while her partner relaxes and fondle and caress her with his hands. There is no magic position right for every body. A suitable position selected from the given diagrams can be selected.

Some people with cancer stop having sex because they fear that it will make the cancer worse. Sometimes it is the vague worry that the sex with a partner suffering from cancer is unclean. A few people believe that a cancer is a punishment for their past sins and try to bargain with God, giving up sex in return for the cancer cure. From a scientific point of view, all these beliefs are not true. The cancer patients can relax and enjoy sex when needed without any bad effects.

Chapter-42

ALLOPATHIC TREATMENT OF CANCER

As stated in the preface of this book, the allopathic treatment or the conventional treatment of cancer is mostly done by the following three methods. These methods are either employed separately or in combination. This chapter has been included in this book, because patients of a homeopathic physician, who when diagnosed with cancer and want to be treated by the conventional methods, ask for the advice of the homoeopath.

RADIATION

This is done by radio-active substances. Radio-active waves are directed at the site of cancer to destroy the cancer cells. Normal or active cells can also be destroyed by this method. It is generally recommended that the patient be prevented from excessive exposure to ionizing radiation. Radiation exposure to the whole body, active blood forming organs, gonads or ocular lens should not increase 5 nems multiplied by the number of years beyond age 18 and that exposure in any 13 consecutive weeks should not exceed 3 nems.

SURGERY

This is a manual operative procedure in which a surgeon removes the cancer or a part of it. In many cases, non-cancerous parts are also removed alongwith the cancerous parts.

CHEMOTHERAPY

Treatment of cancer with anti-cancer chemicals. "Chemo" means chemical and "therapy" means treatment. This method treats the whole patient rather than the specific area. The idea is to wipe out the cancerous cells before they can multiply and form a tumor. One or a number of drugs in combination are used in treatment. Certain hormones such as estrogen are also used. Exactly why they restrict growth of some types of cancer is not completely understood. Alongwith destruction of cancer cells some normal and healthy cells are also destroyed, and this is the main side effect of this type of the treatment. The most affected normal cells are *blood cells, skin cells, hair cells and the cells of the reproductive system.* It is true that some of the side effects are severe but they disappear as soon as the chemotherapy is finished. The most common immediate side effects are nausea and vomiting. The most common late ar delayed side effects are loss of hair, a sore throat, digestive problems, constipation and infections due to blood counts that become lower than the normal. Women may notice changes in their menstrual cycles. The methods of treatment may be oral, injection and intravenous and these rarely cause any pain. There are very few hard and fast rules about the length of treatment because every person is different and every cancer is different. Some chemotherapy affect the kidney and the bladder and hence lots of fluids like water, juices, soups, etc. should be taken during this treatment to keep the kidneys and bladder flushed. Chemotherapy does not affect ability or desire to have sex. One of the waste products of dead cancer cells is uric acid. If the uric acid is allowed to build up in the body, it causes kidney damage or gout. Therefore, alongwith chemotherapy drug\drugs, a medicine is also given to prevent build up of uric acid.

SIDE EFFECTS OF CHEMOTHERAPY	PREVENTION	ACTION BY THE PATIENT
1. More common		
Infections like fever, chills, cough, sore throat. Low white blood cells.	Limit contact with sick people and people suffering from cold. Wash hands often.	If temp. is over 38°C or 100°F, consult the docter immediately.
2. Less common		
a. Bruising or bleeding, black tar-like stools, Red spots on skin—skin rash, gout, swelling of feet and lower legs.	Use sharp objects with care. Inform the doctor before any dental work is done.	If bleeding and bruising is unusual or does not stop, contact the doctor at once.
b. Nausea and vomiting	Drink lot of clear fluids. Get fresh air and rest. Take medicine along with food.	If vomiting lasts for more than 24 hours, contact the doctor.
c. Change in menstrual periods	If as usual, no action is required.	If abnormal, consult the doctor
3. Significant		
Bone loss	This can occur within 6 months of treatment.	Consult the doctor.

4. Rare

Agitation, confusion, seizures, tremors, hallucinations, muscle twitching, shortness of breath, difficulty in walking, yellow eyes or skin and sleeplessness.

Consult the doctor.

NOTE :-

1. Treatment of cancer is a very lengthy process in all the systems of medicines.

2. All the side effects of allopathic treatment can be effectively treated with homoeopathic remedies along with the use of the allopathic medicines. Chemotherapy and other anti-cancer allopathic medicines, etc. are usually to be taken once daily. Indicated homoeopathic remedies for treatment of their side effects, can be taken after about a gap of not less than three hours.

Chapter-43

HOPE FOR THE FUTURE

When a fetus develops and in the process of healing of wounds, the body creates new vessels in the process called *"angiogenesis"* to supply greater amount of blood to the developing tissues. A cancer also needs blood to provide it with oxygen and nutrients as it grows. In cancer cases also, the body develops *"angiogenesis"* to feed the cancer tissues with blood. If the blood supply to the cancer is blocked, the cancer can shrink and die eventually; latest research is being carried out in this direction. In this procedure, an incision of the size of a pencil tip is made into the diseased area and a catheter is guided through an artery to the site of the cancer and small plastic particles are injected into the vessels supplying blood to the cancer. This blocks the vessels and cuts the blood supply to the cancer, causing it to shrink and die. One of the dangers of this procedure can be that the plastic particles may spread in the wrong direction to the other parts of the body causing conditions like blood clots or thrombosis. I hope researchers will find a solution for it.

Y̶ou must have enjoyed going through this book. We at
B. JAIN PUBLISHERS (P) LTD. have many more interesting
topics related to this book. Some of them are as follows:—

THE CURE FOR ALL CANCERS

HULDA REGEHR CLARK

The book includes over 100 case histories of the persons cured. As
new research findings show that there is a single cause for all cancers.
This book provide exact instructions for their cure.

BOOK CODE: BC-5369   PAGES: 650   PRICE: RS. 125.00

CANCER: CAUSE, CARE & CURE

J. BENEDICT D' CASTRO

This book on the cause, care, cure and managemnt of cancer by Dr.
Castro is a concise and complete clinical guide. Cancer, the dreaded
legacy of the 20th century is still unconquerable, even though Modern Medicine has taken giant leaps in the last three decades.

BOOK CODE: BC-5358   PAGES: 350   PRICE: RS. 90.00

CANCER & NUTRITION

CHARLES B. SIMONE

If everyone could read Simone's book early enough in life and take it
seriously, we would make major strides toward putting the cancer
doctors out of work and approach the legacy of health that is within
our reach.

BOOK CODE: BC-3927   PAGES: 338   PRICE: RS. 60.00

B. JAIN PUBLISHERS (P) LTD.
1921, Chuna Mandi, St. 10th Paharganj, New Delhi-110 055
Ph.: 3670572, 3670430, 3683200, 3683300
Fax: 011-3610471 & 3683400
Website: www.bjainbooks. com, Email:bjain@vsnl.com